The Wisdom of Sex...For Men

A Book About Taboo Conversations

By Dr. Heather Wisdom, PsyD LMHC

Dr. Wisdom's YouTube Channel

https://www.youtube.com/@thewisdomof

This book explores the unspoken questions and hidden fears that many men face regarding sex and intimacy - topics that are often difficult to discuss. It provides a non-judgmental space to learn more about these taboo subjects, offering practical insights, advice, and guidance to help men navigate their sexual lives with greater understanding and confidence.

Reading this book straight through will reveal intentional redundancies. This is because many readers may only focus on specific chapters relevant to them. You will find that solutions, exercises, and information are often similar or identical across different topics.

Table of Contents

Introduction: Breaking the Silence

Why Men Need This Book

I understand that for many men, discussing sex, intimacy, and the challenges faced in the bedroom can be really tough. Feeling hesitant due to societal expectations, cultural influences, or personal insecurities is normal. This silence can lead to feelings of isolation and shame.

However, this book is here to help. It's designed to provide men with the tools to break the silence, address unspoken questions, and engage with their sexual experiences more authentically. By delving into these sensitive topics, the book aims to create understanding, self-awareness, and confidence when navigating the complexities of sex and relationships.

Dr. Wisdom's Philosophy

The core of this book is Dr. Wisdom's compassionate approach to men's sexual health, intimacy, and emotional well-being. Dr. Wisdom strongly believes that vulnerability is not a weakness—it's a powerful force for building deeper connections with oneself and one's partner.

Understanding the full spectrum of your emotional, mental, and physical needs is essential for sexual health. This philosophy encourages men to embrace their whole selves, acknowledging their fears, desires, insecurities, and strengths. By doing so, men can achieve a more fulfilling, balanced, and connected experience in their intimate relationships.

The Importance of Honest Conversations

Openly discussing sex is imperative for personal growth and healthy relationships. Honest conversations dispel myths, clarify misunderstandings, reduce anxieties, and foster deeper emotional intimacy. When men feel comfortable discussing their desires, boundaries, and concerns, they not only improve their sexual satisfaction but also enhance their mental health and overall well-being. Starting these conversations may seem daunting, but this book provides practical guidance on initiating and sustaining open, honest dialogues about sex and intimacy. This is not just about communicating with a partner—it's also about developing an internal dialogue with yourself. When you can reflect on your own needs, wants, and fears with honesty and compassion, you pave the way for more fulfilling relationships.

What This Book Offers

In the chapters ahead, we'll be exploring the common challenges that men face in their sexual lives. We'll discuss issues like performance anxiety, erectile dysfunction, emotional disconnect, and navigating desires. Each chapter will offer practical, evidence-based advice and share personal anecdotes in a compassionate, non-judgmental manner to shed light on these experiences.

We'll cover topics like:

- Overcoming the fear of vulnerability
- Dispelling common myths about male sexuality
- How to foster deeper emotional connections with your partner
- Understanding the impact of stress, anxiety, and mental health on sexual performance
- Navigating the complex terrain of sexual desires, fantasies, and boundaries
- The importance of sexual communication, consent, and mutual respect

This journey isn't about achieving perfection; it's about understanding yourself better and building more authentic, satisfying relationships. Sexual fulfillment comes from aligning your physical desires with your emotional and mental well-being, and that starts with having the courage to break the silence.

Let this book serve as your guide as you embark on this journey. By reflecting on your experiences, gaining clarity on your personal needs, and embracing openness, you can reshape how you approach sex and intimacy. While the road ahead may require confronting old habits and deeply held beliefs, it offers a path toward greater wisdom, confidence, and meaningful connection.

Thinkers vs. Feelers – Understanding and Communicating with Different Emotional Processing Styles

Before starting each chapter, it is important to discuss the difference between communicating with a thinker and a feeler. Effective communication is essential in managing relationship issues.

One of the most common sources of misunderstanding in relationships stems from how individuals process emotions. People tend to approach the world as thinkers or feelers, and this distinction can profoundly impact how they communicate, handle conflict, and connect emotionally. Thinkers often prioritize logic, analysis, and problem-solving, while feelers emphasize emotions, intuition, and relationships. Neither approach is right or wrong, but understanding these different processing styles is essential for building strong communication and relationship connections.

This section will explore the key differences between thinkers and feelers, the strengths and challenges of each emotional processing style, and offer practical strategies for communicating effectively with both. If you are a thinker, a feeler, or fall somewhere in between, learning to bridge this divide can lead to deeper understanding, reduced conflict, and more fulfilling relationships.

What Does It Mean to Be a Thinker?

A thinker processes experiences primarily through logic, analysis, and rational thought. Thinkers approach problems in a linear, step-by-step manner, looking for logical solutions and focusing on facts. When confronted with emotional or practical challenges, thinkers often prefer to analyze the situation objectively rather than dive into their feelings. This does not mean that thinkers are emotionless; instead, they tend to compartmentalize emotions in favor of rational thinking, especially regarding decision-making.

Key Characteristics of Thinkers:

<u>Prioritize Logic Over Emotion</u>: Thinkers often value reason and logic above all else. When faced with a problem, they are more likely to ask, "What makes sense?" or "What's the most efficient solution?" rather than focusing on how the situation makes them feel.

<u>Problem-Solvers</u>: Thinkers excel at solving practical problems and approaching challenges rationally. They tend to look for concrete solutions and sometimes become frustrated when emotions complicate the issue.

<u>Objective and Analytical</u>: Thinkers often strive for objectivity, relying on facts and data to inform their decisions. They may distance themselves from emotions when making choices, especially if they believe emotions will cloud their judgment.

<u>Tendency to Compartmentalize Emotions</u>: While thinkers experience emotions, they may not feel comfortable expressing or discussing them openly. Instead, they prefer

to keep their feelings separate from decision-making processes and may view emotional expression as unnecessary or unhelpful.

What Does It Mean to Be a Feeler?

By contrast, a feeler processes experiences primarily through emotions and intuition. Feelers tend to prioritize harmony, relationships, and empathy, focusing on how situations make them feel or how they affect others emotionally. When faced with challenges, feelers are more likely to ask, "How does this make me feel?" or "How will this affect those around me?" Feelers thrive on emotional connection and often seek mutual understanding and emotional resonance in their relationships.

Key Characteristics of Feelers:

Prioritize Emotions Over Logic: Feelers value emotional connection and intuition. When making decisions, they often consider their feelings and the feelings of those around them, sometimes placing emotional well-being above efficiency or practicality.

Empathy and Relationship-Focused: Feelers are deeply attuned to the emotions of others. They often place a high value on relationships and harmony, ensuring everyone feels heard, valued, and understood.

Intuitive and Emotionally Driven: Feelers often rely on their gut instincts and emotional responses when navigating life. They may be more comfortable discussing their emotions and exploring the feelings behind their actions.

<u>Desire for Emotional Expression</u>: Unlike thinkers, feelers are more open about their emotions. They often want to talk about their feelings, process their emotions with others, and seek emotional validation.

Thinkers vs. Feelers: Strengths and Challenges

Both thinkers and feelers bring valuable strengths to relationships, but these different emotional processing styles can also create challenges if not understood and respected.

Strengths of Thinkers:

<u>Logical Decision-Making</u>: Thinkers excel at making rational, well-thought-out decisions, which can be especially helpful in stressful situations where emotions may cloud judgment.

<u>Problem-Solving</u>: Thinkers often approach challenges with clear, actionable steps and can help bring structure to situations that feel overwhelming.

<u>Objectivity</u>: Thinkers' ability to remain objective allows them to view situations without being overly swayed by emotions, providing balance when emotions run high.

Challenges for Thinkers:

<u>Difficulty Expressing Emotions</u>: Thinkers may struggle to open up emotionally, leaving their partners feeling disconnected or frustrated.

<u>Over-Reliance on Logic</u>: In emotionally charged situations, thinkers may overlook the importance of feelings, which can make their partners feel unheard or undervalued.

<u>Avoiding Emotional Conversations</u>: Thinkers may avoid discussing emotions altogether, preferring to focus on facts or solutions, which can create a communication gap in relationships.

Strengths of Feelers:

<u>Emotional Connection</u>: Feelers are often excellent at building emotional intimacy and fostering empathy in relationships. They can help others feel understood and validated.

<u>Relational Awareness</u>: Feelers are highly attuned to the emotional dynamics of their relationships, making them sensitive to mood or emotional needs changes.

<u>Ability to Express Emotions</u>: Feelers are generally more comfortable sharing their emotions, which can help build deeper emotional bonds with their partners.

Challenges for Feelers:

<u>Emotional Decision-Making</u>: Feelers may struggle to make decisions when emotions are involved, sometimes prioritizing feelings over practical solutions.

Difficulty Handling Logic-Driven Conversations: When confronted with a thinker's logical approach, feelers may feel invalidated or dismissed if their emotional needs are not addressed.

Tendency to Over-Emphasize Emotions: Feelers may get caught up in their emotions, sometimes making situations more complicated or overwhelming than necessary.

How to Communicate with a Thinker

If you are a feeler communicating with a thinker, understanding their logical, solution-focused mindset is vital to fostering better communication. Here are some practical tips for effectively engaging with a thinker:

1. Be Direct and Specific

Thinkers appreciate clear, straightforward communication. When discussing an issue, focus on the facts and what you want to achieve. Instead of diving immediately into how you feel, start by outlining the situation logically before bringing in the emotional aspects.

Example: Instead of saying, "I feel really upset that you didn't call me," try saying, "You didn't call me when you said you would, and that hurt me because I thought we had agreed on it."

2. Focus on Solutions, Not Just Emotions

Thinkers often want to solve problems rather than talk about feelings. While expressing your feelings is important, include actionable steps or solutions in the conversation. This helps thinkers feel like they are addressing the issue and can prevent frustration.

<u>Example</u>: Instead of saying, "I feel overwhelmed and don't know what to do," say, "I am overwhelmed, and I think I need help managing my workload. Can we talk about how to handle this together?"

3. Respect Their Need for Space

Thinkers may need time to process their thoughts before responding, especially in emotionally charged situations. Give them the space they need to reflect without pressuring them for an immediate emotional response.

<u>Example</u>: If a thinker seems withdrawn or quiet during an argument, instead of demanding immediate emotional engagement, say, "I understand that you need time to think. Let's revisit this conversation when you're ready."

How to Communicate with a Feeler

Understanding their emotional and relational approach is essential if you are a thinker communicating with a feeler. Feelers often need emotional validation and connection before they can engage in problem-solving. Here are some strategies for engaging effectively with a feeler:

1. Validate Their Emotions

Feelers value emotional connection and validation. Before diving into solutions, acknowledge and validate their feelings. Let them know their emotions are heard and understood, even if you don't fully agree with them.

<u>Example</u>: Instead of immediately offering solutions, try saying, "It sounds like you're feeling really upset. I understand why this is hard for you."

2. Engage in Emotional Conversations

Feelers often need to process their emotions verbally before they're ready to move forward. Be willing to listen and engage in emotional conversations, even if they don't lead directly to a solution.

<u>Example</u>: If a feeler shares their frustrations, listen without interrupting or offering advice. After they've expressed themselves, you can say, "It sounds like this has really been bothering you. How can I support you right now?"

3. Be Open to Emotional Expression

Feelers may want to talk about their emotions openly and frequently, so it's important to be receptive to these conversations. Even if you're uncomfortable with emotional expression, try to create space for these discussions and let them know you're present.

<u>Example</u>: If a feeler wants to talk about their day and how they felt, respond with empathy rather than brushing off their emotions. Say, "I'm here to listen. Tell me more about how you're feeling."

Bridging the Gap: Tips for Harmonious Communication Between Thinkers and Feelers

Successful communication between thinkers and feelers requires empathy, patience, and a willingness to understand each other's processing styles. Here are a few ways to bridge the gap:

1. Acknowledge Each Other's Strengths

Instead of viewing your differences as a source of conflict, acknowledge each approach's strengths to the relationship. Thinkers can help bring clarity and structure to emotionally complex situations, while feelers can provide emotional depth and understanding.

Mutual Respect: Celebrate the fact that thinkers excel at solving problems and navigating challenges with logic, while feelers bring empathy and emotional insight that can enrich the relationship.

2. Compromise and Adaptation

Thinkers and feelers must be willing to adapt and compromise in their communication styles. Thinkers can work on expressing their emotions more openly, while feelers can practice incorporating logic into their emotional discussions.

Example: If you're a thinker, try to focus on your partner's emotions before offering solutions. If you're a feeler, try to present your emotions in a way that also includes a logical component.

3. Use "I" Statements to Reduce Blame

Thinkers and feelers can benefit from using "I" statements to avoid misunderstandings or defensive responses. This approach focuses on expressing one's own perspective without assigning blame to the other person.

<u>Example</u>: Instead of saying, "You never listen to me," say,

Thinker to Feeler: "I *feel* hurt and unheard during our conversations."

Feeler to Thinker: "I *am* hurt and not heard during our conversations."

Understanding and Embracing Emotional Differences

Recognizing the differences between thinkers and feelers is essential for developing stronger emotional and relational bonds. By appreciating each processing style's specific strengths and obstacles, couples can enhance communication, minimize conflicts, and establish more gratifying relationships. Mastery of the art of communication that respects both logic and emotion can effectively bridge the divide between these two emotional realms, regardless of one's inclination towards thinking or feeling.▢

PART I: The Sexual Mind of Men

This section provides a constructive exploration of the psychological and emotional aspects of male sexuality. It sheds light on the often-unspoken fears, desires, and societal pressures that shape men's sexual experiences. By addressing issues like shame, performance anxiety, body image, and emotional intimacy, Part I aims to help men gain a deeper understanding of how their thoughts and beliefs influence their sexual health and relationships. It offers insights and practical tools for building greater self-awareness, confidence, and authentic connections.

Chapter 1: Sexual Shame and Guilt

Sexual shame and guilt can weigh heavily on men, often without expression. These emotions may arise from societal standards, cultural pressures, individual experiences, and religious instruction. This section discusses how these emotions are internalized, how they contribute to performance anxiety, and what steps can be taken to overcome them in a manner that promotes emotional and sexual development.

Internalizing Shame: Societal and Cultural Pressures

Understanding the Roots of Shame:

It's often ingrained in men from a young age that their masculinity should conform to specific societal ideals. They're expected to embody sexual dominance, always be prepared for intimacy, and, above all, never show vulnerability. This pressure can lead men to feel inadequate if they fall short of these unrealistic standards, as society often ties a man's sexual prowess to his value.

In today's society, the confusion surrounding masculinity is compounded by shifting cultural expectations. With the rise of feminist values advocating for gender equality, men are often encouraged to embrace traits traditionally viewed as less masculine—such as emotional openness, gentleness, and active listening. While these changes are central in breaking down harmful stereotypes and promoting equality, they can leave men feeling unsure of their place within modern gender dynamics.

It's really tough for men to navigate the expectations around masculinity. On one hand, they're told to let go of outdated ideas of dominance, but on the other hand, they're still judged by those very same standards. The mixed messages around what it means to be a man can be really confusing. Society expects men to be less aggressive and more sensitive, but at the same time, traditional ideals of the strong, stoic, and assertive alpha male are still glorified in media and social portrayals. This can create a lot of inner conflict and pressure for men, both in their relationships and in society.

Many men struggle with questions about their own masculinity. How can they be emotionally vulnerable without feeling like they're losing their masculinity? How can they support gender equality without feeling emasculated or inadequate? This internal struggle can lead to feelings of alienation, as men try to meet expectations that seem to be constantly changing. It's easy for them to feel like no matter what they do, they're always falling short.

In a world where extreme feminist ideals sometimes call for the rejection of traditional masculinity entirely, men can feel caught in a dilemma: How do they reconcile their natural tendencies with these evolving societal values? Without clear guidance, the result is often confusion, frustration, and a deep sense of uncertainty about how to express their sexuality and masculinity in a healthy, balanced way.

In these confusing and sometimes conflicting societal expectations, it's important for men to find balance and clarity and redefine masculinity on their own terms. Rather than trying to fit into societal molds, men can explore what feels authentic to them. Masculinity doesn't have to conform to rigid ideals of dominance or control—it can also include qualities like compassion, emotional awareness, and adaptability. Modern masculinity is ever-changing, and it's okay to reject extremes and find a balance that suits one's personality and values.

One of the most important changes in societal expectations is the encouragement for men to be more open about their emotions. This openness can be difficult, especially when it contrasts with traditional ideas of masculinity. However, being honest about your feelings, fears, and desires can become a source of strength. It fosters deeper connections with partners, friends, and even yourself. Sharing emotions or admitting uncertainty is not a weakness; it is a meaningful step toward building healthier, more authentic relationships.

Open communication is essential in navigating modern relationships, where gender roles have evolved. Men should feel empowered to discuss their insecurities, desires, and boundaries with their partners. By communicating openly, both men and women can better understand each other's needs and expectations. Instead of feeling pressured to perform according to extreme feminist ideals, men can foster mutual respect and support in their relationships. After all, not all women want a man who conforms to societal feminist ideas.

Addressing societal myths about masculinity is an important step. It's essential for men to question the idea that their worth is tied to sexual performance, dominance, or stoicism. This involves reflecting on the sources of these beliefs—through media, culture, or upbringing—and consciously choosing not to let them dictate self-worth or relationships. Emotional openness is important, but it's equally important for men to establish appropriate boundaries. Embracing vulnerability doesn't mean adhering to a new, inflexible model of sensitivity; men should strive to balance emotional expression with maintaining their sense of self.

It's important to recognize the distinction between men who approach the world as "thinkers" and those who approach it as "feelers." Many men tend to prioritize logic, problem-solving, and analysis, while many women often prioritize emotions, intuition, and relational dynamics. This difference can make it challenging for men to express their emotions openly.

Finding support through therapy, men's groups or friendships can also be helpful. Men can benefit from connecting with others who face similar struggles. Sharing experiences offers clarity, validation, and a sense of community. Openly discussing challenges related to masculinity, relationships, and sex is essential to combat the isolation that often comes with these internal conflicts.

The concept of masculinity is dynamic, and it's important for men to remain open to growth and change. Adapting and evolving as they learn more about themselves and their relationships enables men to navigate these complexities confidently. There is no one-size-fits-all approach—what works today may change over time with new insights and experiences. By promoting open communication, men can develop their version of masculinity that fits them without feeling pressure from external expectations.

Overcoming Sexual Shame:

Sexual shame might stem from doubting your own masculinity, particularly when societal norms set unrealistic expectations for sexual performance and identity. Overcoming this shame involves challenging these external pressures and reshaping your personal connection with your sexuality. This process entails practicing self-compassion, engaging in honest self-examination, and gradually letting go of the myths and stereotypes that surround male sexuality. By embracing a more genuine, personalized comprehension of your desires and experiences, you can start to reclaim your own sexual relationship without judgment.

Exercise 1: for Reframing Shame Around Sexual Performance and Masculinity

1. Identify the Source of Shame

Use a free association technique to reflect on the beliefs you hold about your sexual performance or what it means to be a man. Immediately write down whatever comes to mind without overthinking. It doesn't matter what it is—just put it on paper.

Next, consider where these ideas came from. Were they influenced by media, childhood conversations, cultural expectations, or personal experiences? The goal here is to uncover the sources of any shame or anxiety around sex and masculinity.

<u>Example</u>:

Belief: "I have to perform perfectly in bed, or I'm not a real man."

Source: This belief might come from seeing exaggerated portrayals of male sexual performance in movies or pornography.

2. Challenge the Beliefs

Once you've identified these beliefs, it's time to challenge them. Next to each belief, write a statement that reframes it in a healthier, more realistic way. This step helps break down unrealistic expectations that lead to shame.

<u>Example</u>:

Belief: "I must always be ready for sex, or I'm failing."

Challenged Belief: "Being a man isn't about being 'always on.' It's about connecting with my partner, enjoying the moment, and respecting my own limits."

Challenged Belief: "Desire naturally comes and goes. It's normal not to be in the mood all the time, and that doesn't make me less of a man."

3. Rewrite Your Beliefs About Sex and Masculinity

Now, with the challenged beliefs in mind, write a new narrative for how you see yourself in terms of sex and manhood. Focus on positive and affirming concepts like strength, connection, pleasure, and authenticity. This new narrative should be free from societal pressures and unrealistic expectations, reflecting a more confident and grounded version of yourself.

<u>Example</u>:

New Narrative: "My masculinity is about strength, connection, and mutual respect. I'm not defined by performance, but by the way, I care for my partner and enjoy sex as a shared experience. I allow myself the freedom to feel desire without pressure or guilt."

By completing these exercises, you'll begin shifting your mindset away from external pressures and toward a more authentic, confident understanding of yourself as a man. This process helps to release shame and embrace a healthier, more balanced perspective on sex and masculinity.

Performance Anxiety: The Fear of Not Measuring Up

Why Men Fear Performance Failure:

Many men feel immense pressure to "always perform" at a certain level, believing that their worth as lovers—and even as men—depends on their ability to satisfy their partner in every sexual encounter. This belief is often driven by cultural messages that equate masculinity with sexual prowess, leading men to internalize the idea that any perceived failure in the bedroom reflects a personal inadequacy.

The pressure to perform can create a challenging cycle. When men worry about their ability to perform, it becomes harder to enjoy sex. The mind becomes focused on potential mistakes, outcomes, or insecurities rather than the moment, making it difficult to relax or be fully present with their partner. This mental stress directly affects the body, often manifesting in issues such as erectile dysfunction or premature ejaculation, further reinforcing the belief that they're failing. The fear of failure becomes a self-fulfilling prophecy.

As anxiety increases, the body's natural sexual responses are inhibited. Erections may become difficult to maintain, or ejaculation may happen too quickly due to the overwhelming tension. The more these issues arise, the more men internalize the belief that they are "bad lovers," further compounding their anxiety in future encounters. The result is a cycle where fear leads to anxiety, which leads to physical challenges, which in turn deepens the original fear.

Complicating matters is the fact that men often feel isolated in this struggle. Performance anxiety is rarely discussed openly, and because men are expected to embody strength and confidence, admitting to sexual anxiety can feel like a failure of masculinity. This silence reinforces the shame men feel when they experience difficulties, making it harder to break free from the cycle. They become trapped in a loop of silent suffering, fearing judgment or rejection from their partners if they reveal their anxieties.

This cycle of anxiety is compounded by the expectation of constant readiness. Many men believe they must always be physically prepared for sex, equating masculinity with an endless sexual drive and the ability to perform on demand. This expectation doesn't account for the natural ebb and flow of desire, nor does it acknowledge the mental and emotional factors that contribute to sexual experiences. The pressure to be "always on" means that any deviation from this unrealistic standard is seen as a failure, further reinforcing anxiety.

The good news is that this cycle can be broken. By addressing performance anxiety at its root, men can begin to shift their focus away from unrealistic expectations and toward a healthier, more fulfilling approach to sex. It starts with recognizing that sexual performance does not define worth as a man or a lover. Sex is about connection, mutual enjoyment, and pleasure, not about meeting a set of predefined criteria. When men allow themselves to experience sex as an intimate and fluid process rather than a performance with a set outcome, they can begin to break the hold that anxiety has over them. This shift in mindset opens the door to more relaxed, enjoyable, and satisfying sexual experiences for both partners.

Overcoming Performance Anxiety:

Breaking the cycle of performance anxiety involves shifting focus away from the outcome (e.g., an orgasm or lasting longer) and toward the experience itself. Mindfulness and communication are powerful tools for doing this.

Exercise 2: The 4-6-8 Breathing Technique (A Mindful Approach to Anxiety)

Practice Before Sex: Close your eyes, inhale through your nose for 4 seconds, hold your breath for 6 seconds, and then exhale slowly for 8 seconds through your mouth. Repeat this at least 3 times to relax before sex.

Use During Sex: If you feel anxiety building during sex, pause for a moment and do a shortened version of the exercise (e.g., breathe in for 4 seconds, hold for 4, exhale for 4). This can help refocus your mind on the present *moment.*

When we inhale, our heart rate increases and decreases when we exhale. By practicing these breathing techniques, you engage with your body's relaxation system. This shift helps take your mind off of the performance and bring you back into the moment.

Exercise 3: Sensate Focus (For Men in Relationships)

This is a gradual approach to building sexual connection and removing performance pressure. It emphasizes physical touch and exploration rather than focusing on penetration or orgasm.

Step 1: Non-Sexual Touching: Take turns with your partner touching each other without any expectation of sex. Focus on sensations—warmth, texture, and connection. Communicate openly about what feels good without the goal of arousal.

Step 2: Gradual Re-Introduction of Sexual Touch: Once you both feel comfortable, start incorporating more intimate areas into your touch. Continue to avoid intercourse, focusing purely on pleasure and sensation.

Step 3: Reintroducing Sex: After a few sessions, slowly reintroduce sex. The key here is maintaining the low-pressure approach—sexual connection should feel mutual, without the goal of "performance."

This exercise helps retrain your brain to focus on pleasure and connection, not just on the physical acts of sex or performance. Say things like, "I like that," "I enjoy that," "I like it on the left," and "Move up; that's where I like it." Focusing on what you like and not what you don't like increases confidence.

Navigating Religious and Moral Conflict

The Clash Between Belief and Desire:

Many men grapple with a deep internal struggle as they strive to reconcile their personal or religious beliefs with their natural sexual desires. Growing up in environments where sex is deemed inherently sinful, immoral, or strictly constrained by rules, such as being permissible only within marriage or for procreation, can have a lasting impact. When sexual thoughts and desires emerge, men who hold these beliefs may experience intense guilt or shame, feeling as though their desires are a moral failing. This conflict between their learned beliefs and their natural experiences can create an overwhelming emotional burden.

In many religious and traditional communities, sexual purity is highly valued, and men are often expected to restrain their sexual desires until they meet certain conditions, such as marriage. This can create a strong mental connection between sex and guilt, leading men to feel ashamed even for experiencing normal, healthy sexual urges. Over time, these conflicting emotions can lead men to suppress or deny their sexual needs altogether, believing that acting on or even acknowledging these desires makes them impure or sinful.

It's understandable that because of this repression, men may develop a negative relationship with their sexuality. Instead of seeing sex as a natural part of life, they may perceive it as something to be concealed, controlled, or even eliminated. This can result in feelings of shame, confusion, or self-loathing as they struggle to reconcile their desires with their beliefs. In severe cases, this internal conflict can lead men to perceive themselves as fundamentally flawed or "dirty" for simply having sexual thoughts, which can result in emotional isolation, depression, and anxiety.

The pressure not only affects a man's internal world but can also create significant challenges in relationships. Men who have been taught to associate sex with guilt may find it difficult to openly express their desires with a partner. They might feel hesitant to engage in intimacy, fearing it will compromise their moral integrity. Alternatively, they may act out impulsively, only to feel intense shame afterward. This can create a cycle of emotional distance and sexual dissatisfaction, impacting their well-being and placing strain on their romantic relationships.

The conflict between personal or religious beliefs and sexual desires can lead to self-punishing behaviors in men. Some may choose celibacy or try to excessively control their desires, while others may find themselves in cycles of indulging in sexual behavior followed by deep remorse and self-blame. Unfortunately, this cycle only serves to reinforce feelings of inadequacy, pushing men further into a state of emotional turmoil.

It's important to recognize that this issue can be resolved through time, self-reflection, and empathy. Overcoming these feelings of guilt requires men to dismantle the rigid and often harmful messages they have absorbed about sex. This doesn't mean completely abandoning their personal or religious values, but rather finding a way to incorporate a healthier understanding of sexuality within those belief systems. This process may involve questioning the origins and validity of certain beliefs and acknowledging that sex and desire are natural aspects of being human—not a moral shortcoming.

One-way men can start to address this conflict is by reframing their views on sex. Instead of seeing sexual desire as something inherently bad or shameful, they can learn to view it as a natural expression of their humanity—one that can coexist with their spiritual or moral beliefs. This shift in mindset allows for a more compassionate understanding of sexuality, where desire is acknowledged, accepted, and navigated in a way that aligns with personal values without resulting in guilt or self-condemnation.

Seeking support through therapy, counseling, or discussions with trusted spiritual or community leaders is an essential part of the healing process. Men can explore their beliefs and feelings in a safe and nonjudgmental environment. These conversations can help them find new perspectives, identify where harmful beliefs came from, and learn how to reconcile their desires with their values in a way that promotes emotional and sexual well-being.

Ultimately, finding a balance between personal or religious beliefs and sexual health is a deeply personal journey. For many men, it requires challenging long-held assumptions, letting go of harmful shame, and embracing a more holistic view of themselves. By doing so, they can begin to experience sexual desire not as a source of guilt but as a natural part of their lives, capable of enriching their relationships and personal fulfillment. It's a process of learning to be kind to themselves, recognizing that sexual desires don't define their worth, and finding a way to integrate their beliefs and sexuality in a way that fosters self-acceptance and inner peace.

Finding Peace Between Sexuality and Belief:

It's important to recognize that sexual desire is a natural part of being human. Overcoming this internal conflict means re-examining your beliefs in a way that allows space for both your spirituality and your sexuality.

Exercise 4: Bridging Desire and Belief

Reflect on Your Beliefs: Write down the specific beliefs that are in conflict with your sexual desires. For example, "My religion says that sex outside of marriage is wrong."

Identify What Feels True for You: Examine these beliefs. Do they align with how you truly feel about your sexuality? Is there room in your belief system for growth or reinterpretation? For instance, you might explore if your belief system allows for sexual expression within respectful, consensual relationships.

Talk to a Trusted Mentor or Counselor: Sometimes, working through religious conflicts requires outside perspective. Consider seeking a therapist who specializes in sexual health and spirituality or a trusted religious mentor who takes an open-minded approach. Having an external viewpoint can help you navigate this complex terrain.

By integrating your desires with your personal values, you can ease the internal conflict and move toward a more holistic and fulfilling sexual life that aligns with your beliefs.

Releasing Guilt and Embracing a New Narrative

Sexual shame and guilt are not flaws in your character—they are burdens imposed by external expectations. Releasing them requires compassion, mindfulness, and a willingness to redefine what sexuality means to you. By challenging societal norms, practicing mindfulness to combat performance anxiety, and finding peace between your beliefs and desires, you can start to build a more authentic and fulfilling sexual life.

Bonus Tip: Journaling as a Daily Practice

After each exercise, take 5 minutes to journal your thoughts. Write about how the exercises made you feel—what emotions came up, what you learned, and what you want to work on next. This small daily practice can help cement progress and bring clarity to areas where you still feel conflicted.

Chapter 2: The Silent Struggle: Why Men Fear Sexual Rejection

Sexual rejection can be an extremely vulnerable and emotionally charged experience for men. It can deeply affect self-esteem, leading to feelings of inadequacy, insecurity, and shame. For many, the fear of rejection is not only about the physical act itself but also about what it represents – an unspoken judgment on their desirability, masculinity, or worth. Despite its common occurrence, the fear of rejection is seldom openly discussed, leaving many men to grapple with it in silence.

In this chapter, we will discuss the origins of this fear and its impact on self-esteem and provide practical strategies to reframe rejection as a natural part of a healthy sexual and emotional life. By addressing rejection constructively, men can develop greater resilience, build sexual confidence, and foster deeper, more meaningful relationships.

Understanding the Roots of Fear and Why It May Feel So Personal

The fear of rejection is deeply ingrained in our biological and social instincts. Throughout evolution, humans have been programmed to seek acceptance, approval, and a sense of belonging, especially in close relationships. Rejection can be perceived as a threat to one's social status, identity, or even survival, particularly when it's related to reproduction and partnership.

For men, this fear is often intensified by cultural norms and societal expectations that link male value to sexual conquest and performance. From a young age, boys are taught to see sexual success as a fundamental aspect of their masculinity. The pressure to excel sexually can make rejection feel like a failure, not just in the moment, but as a reflection of one's overall masculinity.

Men often feel the pressure to always be in control, both physically and emotionally. When they experience rejection, they can feel powerless and exposed. Rejection can make men feel undesired or like they're not good enough. This can lead to a loss of self-confidence over time, causing them to become hesitant in initiating intimacy and expressing their desires, ultimately limiting their emotional and sexual experiences.

The Silent Impact on Self-Esteem

Rejection can be deeply painful and can have long-lasting effects on a man's self-esteem. Over time, being rejected repeatedly can lead to a belief that one is unattractive, incapable, or unworthy of love and intimacy. Even when rejection is not a reflection of personal inadequacy, men may internalize it as proof that something is inherently wrong with them.

Many men respond to rejection with shame. They may feel embarrassed for misreading a situation, for wanting something their partner doesn't want, or for simply being turned down. They may also feel anger toward themselves and the person who rejected them. This anger can manifest in various ways such as lashing out, withdrawing emotionally, or turning to unhealthy coping mechanisms like substance use or promiscuity in an attempt to regain a sense of power and control.

These feelings can cause men to emotionally withdraw, distancing themselves from their partners and from future intimate experiences in an effort to protect their self-esteem. Unfortunately, this only reinforces feelings of isolation, unworthiness, and disconnection.

Rejection is Not Personal: Reframing the Experience

One of the key steps in overcoming the fear of rejection is to reframe it in a healthier, more constructive way. It's important to understand that rejection doesn't always reflect on you as a person, your attractiveness, or your sexual abilities. Most of the time, rejection is about compatibility, timing, or personal boundaries that are unrelated to your worth as a lover or partner.

Consider these reframing perspectives:

Rejection Reflects the Other Person's Needs or Preferences: Everyone has different needs, desires, and boundaries when it comes to sex and intimacy. Rejection often reflects the other person's feelings or circumstances at the moment rather than a judgment on your attractiveness or abilities. It's important to understand that someone's lack of interest may have more to do with where they are emotionally, physically, or mentally than it does with you.

<u>Sexual Rejection Isn't a Rejection of You as a Whole</u>: Sexual rejection often feels deeply personal because sex is such an intimate and vulnerable act. However, just because someone isn't in the mood for sex or doesn't feel the same level of attraction doesn't mean they reject you as a person. People can still value, care for, and appreciate you even if they're not interested in sex at a given moment.

<u>Rejection is a Normal Part of Human Experience</u>: Everyone experiences rejection at some point, in both romantic and non-romantic contexts. It's a normal part of life. By recognizing that rejection is an inevitable part of relationships, you can begin to see it as a shared human experience rather than a unique failure.

<u>Rejection Offers an Opportunity for Growth</u>: Rather than seeing rejection as a negative outcome, try to view it as an opportunity to grow and learn. Rejection can provide insights into your desires, boundaries, and emotional needs and how you navigate intimacy with others. It can also teach you how to handle disappointment with grace and resilience, ultimately making you more confident and secure in future encounters.

Practical Strategies for Handling Rejection Constructively

Dealing with rejection in a healthy way requires both emotional resilience and practical tools to navigate difficult moments. Here are some steps to handle rejection constructively:

1. Normalize Rejection

Remind yourself that rejection is a part of life, not an indictment of your worth. Everyone gets rejected at some point. By normalizing rejection, you can begin to reduce its emotional sting and see it as part of the broader landscape of human relationships.

2. Don't Internalize It

When you experience rejection, resist the urge to internalize it as a judgment on your desirability or masculinity. Instead, focus on the external factors that might be influencing the situation. Was the timing off? Was your partner stressed or tired? Did the rejection reflect something about their emotional state rather than your desirability?

3. Practice Emotional Detachment

It's important to detach your sense of self-worth from sexual validation. While it's natural to feel disappointment or sadness after being rejected, try not to let it define how you see yourself. Practice reminding yourself that you are valuable, worthy, and attractive—regardless of any single experience of rejection.

4. Communicate Openly

After being rejected, it's helpful to have an open and honest conversation with your partner (if applicable) to understand their feelings and needs. Communication can help clear up misunderstandings, reduce feelings of uncertainty, and foster deeper emotional intimacy. Remember that discussing rejection isn't about blaming or demanding validation—it's about understanding your partner's perspective and finding ways to connect more meaningfully.

5. Build Sexual Confidence

One of the most powerful ways to combat the fear of rejection is to build your sexual confidence. This comes from embracing your body, understanding your sexual desires, and focusing on the connection you share with your partner rather than on specific outcomes. Confidence grows when you shift your mindset from one of performance to one of mutual pleasure and exploration.

6. Practice Self-Compassion

Rejection can feel painful, but it's important to practice self-compassion and treat yourself with kindness during these moments. Avoid negative self-talk and focus on affirming your worth. Recognize that it's okay to feel disappointed or hurt, but these feelings don't define who you are.

Building Resilience: The Power of Persistence

Overcoming the fear of rejection is not about avoiding rejection altogether—because that's impossible. Instead, it's about building resilience so rejection doesn't devastate your confidence or self-esteem. Developing resilience requires a willingness to face rejection head-on and keep moving forward, knowing rejection is part of the process.

Every experience of rejection can be difficult, but it's also an opportunity to strengthen your emotional foundation and build a deeper sense of self-worth. By learning to navigate rejection without letting it control your actions, you can cultivate persistence, adaptability, and a growth mindset. This resilience will not only improve your sexual confidence but also enhance all areas of your life.

Rejection and Relationships: Fostering Understanding

Experiencing rejection in romantic relationships can be tough. It's completely normal to face rejection from time to time due to differences in sex drive, stress, or emotional disconnection. Learning how to handle rejection in a positive way is important for maintaining a healthy, honest, and respectful relationship.

Couples who openly communicate about their needs and boundaries, without making each other feel guilty or inadequate, are better equipped to deal with rejection without it causing conflict or resentment. In a committed relationship, having open discussions about rejection can help both partners feel more secure, respected, and valued, even when they're not on the same page sexually.

Exercises to Build Resilience Against Rejection

Exercise 1: Rejection Reframing Practice

Reflect on a time when you experienced rejection (sexual or otherwise).

Write down how it made you feel and what thoughts came up about yourself during the experience.

Now, reframe the rejection by writing a more objective narrative. Focus on external factors, such as timing or the other person's needs, and avoid self-blame.

End by writing a positive affirmation about your worth unrelated to the rejection.

Exercise 2: Build Emotional Buffer Zones

After a rejection, give yourself time to process it without reacting impulsively. Engage in activities that help you feel grounded, like going for a walk, meditating, or journaling.

Use this time to remind yourself of your positive qualities and strengths, reinforcing your self-worth without relying on external validation.

Exercise 3: Confidence Affirmation Practice

Create a Personal Mantra: Develop a mantra that speaks to your value beyond sex. It could be something like, "I am worthy of love and connection, regardless of my partner's desire in the moment."

Or maybe a more realistic one for some; "I'm Ok, my partner loves me even if my she doesn't want me right now."

Repeat It Daily: Say this mantra every morning or after any instance of rejection. Over time, this builds a mindset that internalizes confidence, even when things don't go as expected.

Reconnecting With Your Body

Sexual rejection can make you feel disconnected from your own body. Engaging in activities that help you reconnect physically can boost confidence and reduce negative thoughts about rejection.

Exercise 4: Physical Confidence Routine

Daily Movement: Incorporate 10-15 minutes of daily physical activity, like stretching, yoga, or light exercise. Moving your body not only releases endorphins but also helps you feel more connected and confident in your own skin.

Self-Exploration: Spend time getting to know your body through self-touch that isn't focused on masturbation. Running your hands over your skin, massaging tense areas, and focusing on how your body feels can increase comfort and confidence in your body.

Posture Practice: Improving posture has a direct impact on how you feel about yourself. Stand tall, roll your shoulders back, and take up space—this naturally boosts confidence and can subtly shift how you feel when facing sexual rejection.

Cultivating Emotional Resilience

Facing rejection with resilience means developing the ability to bounce back without internalizing it as a failure. This requires a shift in how you view rejection and your role in the relationship.

Exercise 5: The 3-to-1 Reframe

After Rejection, Write Down 3 Positive Things About Your Relationship: For every rejection, reflect on three positive aspects of your relationship or your partner's love for you. It could be things like, "We communicate well" or "She shows love in non-sexual ways."

Acknowledge Your Partner's Love Languages: Understand that sexual rejection doesn't mean rejection of the relationship. If your partner shows affection in other ways (such as through touch, words of affirmation, or acts of service), take note of this. It reinforces that rejection in one area doesn't mean a lack of love or desire overall.

Celebrate Small Wins: Building resilience also involves celebrating moments of intimacy that don't involve sex. Did you have a deep conversation? Did your partner hold your hand? Acknowledge and celebrate these acts of connection.

Embracing Rejection as Part of Growth

Fear of rejection is a powerful force, but it doesn't have to control your life. By reframing rejection as part of the human experience, practicing emotional resilience, and building self-compassion, you can learn to face rejection with greater confidence and strength. Each experience of rejection is an opportunity to grow—both as an individual and in your relationships.

Embrace the reality that rejection is part of the journey toward deeper connections, both sexually and emotionally. When you no longer fear rejection, you open the door to richer, more fulfilling relationships and a more authentic, empowered sense of self.

□

Chapter 3: Body Image Insecurities

Body image issues are often seen as a "women's problem," but many men silently struggle with feelings of inadequacy about their bodies. These insecurities can deeply impact self-esteem, relationships, and sexual confidence. In this chapter, we'll explore the hidden world of men's body image concerns, how societal pressures shape these insecurities, and actionable strategies for reclaiming body confidence.

Men's Hidden Body Image Issues: Feeling Inadequate but Staying Silent

The societal conditioning that shapes men's perspectives on body image starts at a young age, deeply ingrained in the messages boys receive from parents, peers, media, and culture. From early childhood, boys are often encouraged to "toughen up" and suppress emotions that may be perceived as weak or vulnerable. This expectation doesn't just apply to how boys handle their emotions—it extends to how they perceive and present their bodies. The idea that a man's worth is tied to his physical appearance and strength is pervasive, with societal norms equating masculinity with physical dominance, muscularity, and stoicism.

As boys transition into manhood, these early lessons become ingrained in their internal dialogue. Society expects men to display unwavering confidence, strength, and self-reliance—traits often linked to traditional masculinity.

Conversations about body insecurities are viewed as conflicting with this image, reinforcing the notion that men should be both physically and emotionally self-sufficient. Acknowledging struggles with body image—whether it's feeling too thin, too heavy, not muscular or tall enough, or coping with hair loss—can feel like a direct challenge to this deeply rooted narrative of toughness and control.

The Pressure to Avoid Vulnerability

A central aspect of this struggle is men's pressure to avoid any sign of vulnerability. Society often perceives this as a weakness in men, and since body image concerns are closely linked to feelings of insecurity and inadequacy, they remain a taboo subject. Men are expected to project confidence, power, and control in every aspect of life, including physical appearance. Admitting to body insecurities is often seen as a loss of control, which clashes with these deeply ingrained societal expectations.

For many men, admitting that they're dissatisfied with their bodies feels like a personal failure—a failure to meet not only societal expectations but also their own internalized standards. This can lead to a sense of isolation, as men may believe they're the only ones struggling with these issues. The fear of judgment or ridicule prevents them from seeking support, and in many cases, they may not even realize that other men feel the same way. This creates a culture of silence around men's body image issues, where the pressure to conform is felt but never openly discussed.

The Emotional Consequences of Silence

The silence surrounding men's body image concerns can have serious emotional consequences. When men are unable to express their insecurities, they're left to internalize their feelings, which can lead to shame, self-loathing, or depression. The more men feel they fall short of societal expectations, the more they may begin to view themselves as unworthy or inadequate. This negative self-perception can spill over into other areas of life, affecting relationships, career ambitions, and overall mental health.

Feelings of shame around body image can also lead men to withdraw from intimate relationships or avoid social situations where their bodies are exposed, such as swimming, working out in a gym, or even dating. This isolation only deepens the emotional impact, as it reinforces the belief that they are "not enough" and that their bodies are something to be hidden rather than accepted or celebrated. Over time, this can contribute to anxiety, low self-esteem, and even a sense of hopelessness as men struggle to reconcile their self-image with societal ideals.

Moreover, the pressure to remain silent about these issues can make it difficult for men to seek the help they need. While women may feel more comfortable discussing their body image struggles with friends or seeking therapy, men are often reluctant to do so for fear of being perceived as weak or less masculine. This reluctance to seek help compounds the problem, leaving men trapped in a cycle of self-criticism and silence.

Expanding the Narrative of Masculinity

To break this silence, it's essential to broaden the definition of masculinity to include self-compassion, emotional openness, and the ability to seek support. Men should feel comfortable expressing insecurities without fear of judgment. Body image concerns are not a sign of weakness but a shared human experience that affects both men and women. By challenging societal norms and fostering open conversations about these topics, men can start to redefine masculinity, embracing a more inclusive and healthier sense of self-worth that goes beyond physical appearance.

In breaking this silence, men can develop a more positive and realistic relationship with their bodies, one that recognizes the value of health, strength, and individuality over rigid societal standards. It's time to shift the focus from the external pressures of perfection to the internal acceptance of one's body as unique, capable, and worthy, regardless of how it compares to unrealistic ideals.

Exercise 1: Bringing Your Insecurities to Light

This exercise is designed to help you confront your hidden body insecurities and reframe them more positively.

Identify Your Body Insecurities: Take a few minutes to write down specific aspects of your body that you feel insecure about. Be as honest as possible, masculinity it's your weight, muscle tone, height, or even hair loss.

Ask Where These Insecurities Came From: Next to each insecurity, write down where this belief originated. Was it something you saw in the media, a comment someone made, or societal expectations? This will help you recognize that many of these beliefs are externally imposed.

Reframe Each Insecurity: Challenge each insecurity by writing a neutral or positive statement about that part of your body. For example, if you wrote, "I feel ashamed of my stomach," reframe it as, "My stomach is a part of me, and it doesn't define my worth."

Muscle Dysmorphia and Appearance Pressure

Muscle dysmorphia is characterized by an intense preoccupation with not being muscular enough, even when the person is already highly muscular. This distorted body image leads men to feel that they are never "big" or "lean" enough, which often results in excessive exercising, strict dieting, and the use of supplements or anabolic steroids to try to achieve their ideal physique. Despite achieving visible muscularity, men with muscle dysmorphia continue to feel dissatisfied with their appearance.

The Pressure to Be "Muscular" or "Fit":

One of the most pervasive body image issues that men face is the pressure to be muscular and fit. From advertising to media portrayals, cultural norms continually glorify the "ideal" male body—lean, muscular, and powerful. Men are constantly bombarded with images of superhero physiques in movies, fitness influencers on social media, or athletic role models, that set an unrealistic standard for how they should look.

This societal pressure can lead to a condition known as muscle dysmorphia, where men are never satisfied with their muscle size or definition, no matter how much they work out. As a result, they may engage in excessive exercise routines, obsess over strict diets, or resort to dangerous practices like anabolic steroid use to achieve their desired physique. Unfortunately, this pursuit of the "perfect" body can overshadow personal health and well-being, causing both physical harm and mental distress.

The Harmful Cycle of Comparison

One of the major obstacles to body confidence is the tendency to compare yourself to others. In today's world, where social media showcases perfectly curated images of people's lives and bodies, it's easy to fall into the trap of measuring your worth based on what others look like. The problem with comparison is that it often leads to feelings of inadequacy, as you're likely comparing yourself to an idealized, edited version of someone else's life that doesn't reflect reality.

To break this cycle, it's important to reduce your exposure to unrealistic portrayals of bodies—especially on social media. Consider curating your feed to include content that promotes body positivity, health, and individuality rather than an unattainable standard of perfection. Taking breaks from social media or limiting your time spent scrolling can also help reset your perspective and give you the mental space to focus on your own body and life.

Additionally, practicing gratitude for your body's unique qualities can help diminish the power of comparison. Every body is different, and what works for one person might not work for another. By appreciating your body for what it is and recognizing its strengths, you can stop comparing yourself to others and focus on your own journey toward health and well-being.

Setting personal, non-aesthetic goals can also help you shift your mindset away from comparison. Rather than focusing on how your body looks, focus on what it can achieve. Setting functional goals helps you create a sense of accomplishment that isn't tied to appearance. For example, improving your stamina, increasing your strength, or enhancing your mental clarity through exercise. When you focus on your body's performance and abilities, you'll naturally build more confidence as you witness your progress over time.

Exercise 2: Breaking the Comparison Cycle

This exercise helps break the habit of comparing your body to others and shifts the focus back to your own well-being.

Limit Social Media Exposure: For one week, reduce or limit your exposure to fitness influencers or body-related content on social media. Reflect on how this makes you feel. Do you notice a change in how you perceive your body when you're not constantly comparing it to others?

Practice Gratitude for Your Body: Each morning, write down one thing about your body that you're grateful for. This could be its strength, resilience, or its ability to support you through daily activities. Shifting focus to what your body can do helps reframe how you view it.

Set Personal, Non-Aesthetic Goals: Instead of focusing on appearance-based goals (e.g., "I want bigger biceps"), set performance-related goals (e.g., "I want to lift a certain amount of weight" or "I want to improve my stamina"). This shifts the focus from how your body looks to how it performs and feels.

Reclaiming Control: Steps Toward Body Confidence

Body image insecurities can feel overwhelming, but they don't have to control your self-esteem or your life. Understanding where these insecurities originate and how societal pressures influence them is the first step toward breaking free from their grip. When you identify the sources of these anxieties—childhood experiences, media portrayals, or societal norms—you can begin to unravel their hold over you.

Reclaiming a confident relationship with your body involves shifting your mindset from external validation to internal acceptance. This process requires you to challenge the messages you've internalized over the years and actively create new, healthier narratives. Instead of focusing on achieving an idealized version of your body—one that aligns with impossible standards set by media or cultural expectations—you can begin to focus on what your body does for you, how it supports your life, and how you can care for it holistically.

Body Neutrality: Shifting the Focus from Appearance to Function

Practicing body neutrality is one powerful approach to overcoming insecurities. Body neutrality isn't about loving every part of your body unconditionally; instead, it's about accepting your body as it is without attaching your self-worth to its appearance. The idea is to shift the focus from what your body looks like to what it can do for you on a daily basis. Your body enables you to live, move, work, and connect with others. By recognizing these functional aspects, you can start to appreciate your body for its abilities rather than its aesthetics.

For example, instead of criticizing your arms for not being muscular enough, appreciate them for their strength and ability to lift, carry, and help you engage with the world around you. Instead of fixating on your weight or stomach size, focus on how your body supports your overall health and vitality. This shift from aesthetics to functionality helps you build a healthier relationship with your body, one that isn't dominated by negative self-talk.

Body neutrality allows you to view your body as a vehicle for life, one that doesn't need to look a certain way to be worthy of care and respect. This approach reduces the pressure to constantly monitor and critique your appearance, fostering a more balanced and peaceful relationship with your physical self.

Exercise 3: Body Neutrality Practice

Practice Mirror Work: Stand in front of a mirror and observe your body. Instead of focusing on perceived flaws, try to remain neutral. For example, instead of saying, "I hate my stomach," reframe it as, "This is my stomach. It digests my food and gives me energy." Practicing body neutrality means focusing on the function of your body rather than its appearance.

Celebrate Small Wins: Acknowledge every small victory your body achieves, such as completing a workout, taking a long walk, or simply getting out of bed on a tough day. This helps reinforce the idea that your body's value lies in what it can do, not how it looks.

Building a Positive Body Image Through Movement

True body confidence comes from embracing your body's functionality and health rather than its external appearance. This means shifting your focus from superficial goals like having a six-pack or reaching a certain weight to more meaningful objectives like feeling energized, sleeping better, or improving your strength and mobility. When you prioritize health and functionality, you can begin to appreciate your body for all it allows you to do rather than how it looks in a mirror or a photograph.

Focusing on your health doesn't just mean engaging in physical activity. It also involves taking care of your mental and emotional well-being. Eating nourishing foods, getting enough sleep, practicing mindfulness, and managing stress are necessary to a healthy lifestyle. When you take care of your body holistically—physically, mentally, and emotionally—you're reinforcing the idea that your worth isn't tied to appearance but to your overall well-being.

This holistic approach can also help you break free from the all-or-nothing mindset often accompanying body insecurities. Instead of focusing on achieving a perfect body, you can focus on incremental, sustainable changes supporting your overall health. Small daily actions—like drinking more water, going for a walk, or practicing mindfulness—can profoundly impact your sense of well-being. As you cultivate healthier habits, you'll feel more empowered in your body, regardless of how it looks.

Exercise should be a way to celebrate your body's abilities, not a punishment for not looking a certain way. By shifting your mindset around movement, you can begin to associate exercise with joy and health rather than appearance and aesthetics.

Exercise 4: Joyful Movement

Find a Physical Activity You Enjoy: Choose an exercise you genuinely enjoy, (swimming, hiking, yoga) not for appearance but for how it makes you feel. Focus on how your body feels during and after the activity.

Track How You Feel, Not How You Look: Write down how the exercise made you feel after each session. Did you feel more energetic? More connected to your body? Did it help reduce stress? Shifting the focus from aesthetics to wellness helps redefine your relationship with exercise and your body.

Embracing Individuality

No two bodies are the same, and that's something to celebrate. Your body is unique, with its own characteristics, strengths, and challenges. Part of building body confidence is learning to embrace the features that make you distinct. Your body has its own story. Your height, muscle structure, skin tone, and metabolism are unique to you. Comparing it to someone else's will never do it justice.

Embracing your individuality means rejecting the idea that there is a one-size-fits-all standard of beauty or fitness. Instead of striving to fit into someone else's mold, you can learn to appreciate the aspects of your body that make you different. This shift in perspective helps you cultivate self-acceptance and allows you to see your body as something that is inherently valuable, simply because it is yours.

As you practice self-acceptance, you'll begin to develop a deeper sense of self-worth that isn't tied to external validation or societal expectations. This inner confidence allows you to move through life with a greater sense of freedom and authenticity. By celebrating your individuality, you free yourself from the pressures of conformity and open the door to a more positive and empowered relationship with your body.

Exercise 5: Appreciation Journaling

Daily Body Appreciation: Each day, write down one thing you appreciate about your body. It could be something functional like, "I'm grateful for my legs because they allow me to walk," or something aesthetic like, "I like how strong my shoulders look today." Focusing on appreciation helps you gradually become more confident in your body's abilities and appearance.

Embracing a New Perspective on Body Confidence

True body confidence isn't about achieving a "perfect" body—it's about accepting and celebrating the body you have, with all its imperfections, strengths, and uniqueness. By focusing on health, functionality, and individuality, you can develop a positive, empowered relationship with your body that goes beyond superficial appearance. Confidence comes from within and grows as you learn to appreciate your body for what it does rather than how it looks.

To achieve this, you must be willing to challenge societal norms, break the comparison cycle, and shift your focus to what truly matters—your health, well-being, and individuality. This process takes time, patience, and self-compassion, but the result is a deeper sense of self-worth and a more fulfilling relationship with your body.

By embracing your body for all it is—capable, resilient, and unique—you can reclaim control over your self-esteem and live with greater confidence and authenticity. You have the power to reshape how you see yourself, and it starts with understanding that your worth is not defined by your appearance but by the strength, health, and life your body allows you to experience.

PART II: The Physical Challenges

While emotional and psychological factors play a significant role in men's sexual and intimate lives, physical challenges also contribute to their experiences and overall satisfaction. From concerns about sexual performance to body image issues, these physical challenges can impact self-esteem, relationships, and well-being. In this part of the book, we will explore the most common physical issues men face and offer practical solutions for overcoming them. By addressing these challenges head-on, men can foster a healthier relationship with their bodies and enjoy more fulfilling sexual experiences.

Chapter 4: Erectile Dysfunction and Other Sexual Performance Issues

Erectile dysfunction (ED) is often portrayed as an issue that only affects older men, but the reality is far more complex. Many men, regardless of age, experience challenges related to sexual performance at some point in their lives. The stigma surrounding ED, especially for younger men, can lead to silence, shame, and anxiety, making it harder to address the problem head-on. This chapter focuses on breaking the silence around ED, exploring why it's increasingly common in younger men, and offering non-medical approaches to managing and overcoming it.

Understanding Erectile Dysfunction: More Than Just a Physical Problem

Erectile dysfunction is typically defined as the inability to achieve or maintain an erection firm enough for sexual intercourse. While ED can have physiological causes—such as blood flow problems, hormonal imbalances, or neurological issues—it's important to recognize that sexual performance is also heavily influenced by psychological, emotional, and relational factors.

For many men, sexual performance is tied to their sense of masculinity, self-worth, and character. When ED occurs, it can feel like a personal failure, triggering a range of emotions like frustration, embarrassment, guilt, and shame. These feelings are often compounded by societal expectations that men should always be "ready" for sex, leading to heightened performance anxiety. As a result, ED is rarely just a physical issue—it's a multifaceted challenge that involves mental, emotional, and relational components.

The Rise of ED in Younger Men

ED Isn't Just an "Old Man's Problem" Anymore:

One of the biggest myths about erectile dysfunction is that it only affects older men. However, ED is on the rise among younger men, particularly those in their 20s and 30s. A number of modern-day stressors and lifestyle factors drive this trend.

Although erectile dysfunction is more commonly associated with aging, there has been a notable increase in ED among younger men in recent years. This rise in younger men experiencing ED highlights the importance of understanding that sexual performance issues aren't just a product of aging—they can be triggered by a variety of lifestyle, psychological, and relational factors.

Causes of ED in Younger Men

Psychological Factors:

Performance Anxiety: One of the most common causes of ED in younger men is performance anxiety. The pressure to perform well in bed, particularly with new partners, can create a cycle of anxiety and self-doubt, making it difficult to relax and enjoy the experience. When men feel as though they must always perform at a certain level, this anxiety can interfere with their ability to achieve and maintain an erection.

<u>Depression and Mental Health</u>: Mental health conditions like depression, anxiety, and stress can have a direct impact on sexual performance. These conditions can alter brain chemistry, decrease libido, and make it harder for men to focus on pleasure and connection during sex.

<u>Pornography Use and Unrealistic Expectations</u>: The widespread availability of pornography has created a generation of men who may have unrealistic expectations about what sex should look and feel like. Over time, frequent pornography consumption can desensitize men to real-life sexual experiences, creating difficulties in achieving arousal or satisfaction during partner sex.

Lifestyle Factors:

<u>Stress and Fatigue</u>: Younger men often juggle demanding careers, social obligations, and personal goals, leading to chronic stress and fatigue. Both can significantly impact sexual performance, as high-stress levels increase cortisol production, which inhibits testosterone and affects libido.

<u>Poor Diet and Lack of Exercise</u>: A sedentary lifestyle, poor diet, and lack of exercise can all contribute to erectile dysfunction. These factors can lead to weight gain, decreased cardiovascular health, and reduced blood flow, all of which are critical to maintaining an erection.

<u>Alcohol and Substance Use</u>: Excessive alcohol or drug use can also contribute to ED. Alcohol is a depressant that can interfere with sexual arousal and performance, while recreational drugs may alter mood, impair judgment, and reduce physical functioning.

Relational Factors:

<u>Relationship Issues</u>: Problems in a relationship—communication, trust, or emotional connection—can also contribute to erectile dysfunction. When a man feels emotionally disconnected or insecure in a relationship, it may manifest physically during sexual encounters.

<u>Fear of Rejection</u>: A fear of sexual rejection can lead to ED, particularly if a man is unsure about his partner's level of attraction or satisfaction. This fear can cause anxiety, making it difficult to achieve or maintain an erection.

Breaking the Silence Around Erectile Dysfunction

The stigma surrounding erectile dysfunction often prevents men from seeking help or talking openly about their struggles. Many men feel ashamed or embarrassed by their inability to perform sexually, viewing it as a personal failing rather than a common and treatable issue. However, breaking the silence around ED is a vital step toward addressing the problem.

Challenging the Stigma

<u>ED is Common</u>: One of the first steps in overcoming the shame of ED is recognizing that it is a common experience for men of all ages. Research shows that as many as 40% of men will experience some form of ED by the time they reach 40, and rates are rising among younger men due to lifestyle, psychological, and relational factors.

<u>ED Doesn't Define Your Masculinity</u>: Erectile dysfunction doesn't define your masculinity, worth, or ability to be a loving, intimate partner. Just as men can have good or bad days in other areas of life, sexual performance can vary due to stress, fatigue, or emotional factors. It's important to separate your sexual performance from your overall identity as a man.

<u>Open Conversations with Partners</u>: One of the best ways to address ED is to open up to your partner about what you're experiencing. Many men fear that their partner will be disappointed or frustrated, but in reality, most partners appreciate honesty and will be supportive. By discussing your concerns and exploring other ways to experience intimacy and pleasure, you can reduce the pressure on "performing" and focus on connection.

Why It's Okay to Talk About It:

The key to overcoming ED is recognizing that it's a health issue like any other. Talking about it with a partner, a doctor, or a therapist can be incredibly empowering. When men break the silence, you often discover you aren't alone—and that solutions exist. Bringing ED into the light normalizes it and reduces the fear and shame that often surrounds it.

Exercise 1: Speaking Up About ED

Start with Yourself: If you're struggling with ED, the first step is acknowledging it without judgment. Write down your feelings about ED—are you frustrated, embarrassed, or confused? Getting these emotions out on paper helps you clarify your thoughts.

Open a Conversation with Your Partner: A simple, calm conversation with your partner can alleviate much of the tension. Try saying something like, "I've noticed some changes in my body, and it's been affecting my performance. I'd love to work on this together." This opens the door to communication without blaming yourself or your partner.

Talk to a Professional: If talking to a partner feels intimidating or you're not sure where to start, consult a healthcare provider or therapist who specializes in sexual health. They can provide professional advice and support without judgment.

Exercise 2: Reducing Stress and Anxiety for Better Performance

Practice Daily Relaxation: Incorporate stress-reducing activities like yoga, meditation, or deep breathing into your routine. Even 10 minutes a day can lower cortisol levels and reduce anxiety around sex.

Create a Pre-Sex Routine: If performance anxiety is a concern, create a calming routine before sex. This could include breathing exercises, listening to soothing music, or engaging in non-sexual physical affection to ease the pressure of performance.

Mindful Masturbation: Reduce reliance on pornography by practicing mindful masturbation. This involves focusing on sensation and pleasure rather than visual stimulation or fantasy. It helps retrain your brain to respond to real-life sexual stimuli.

Non-Medical Approaches to Managing Erectile Dysfunction

While there are various medical treatments for ED, such as medications, pumps, or surgery, many men can benefit from addressing the root causes of their performance issues through non-medical approaches. These strategies focus on improving mental, emotional, and relational well-being, as well as making lifestyle changes that support overall sexual health.

1. Mindfulness and Relaxation Techniques

Mindfulness is a powerful tool for managing anxiety and stress, both of which contribute to ED. By practicing mindfulness, men can focus on the present moment and cultivate a deeper sense of awareness and relaxation during sexual experiences.

Breathing Exercises: Controlled breathing can help reduce performance anxiety by slowing the heart rate and calming the nervous system. Deep, slow breaths before and during sexual activity can help ease tension and improve focus on pleasure rather than performance.

<u>Sensate Focus Therapy</u>: This therapeutic approach encourages couples to explore non-sexual touch as a way to build intimacy and reduce performance pressure. By removing the expectation of intercourse, men can relax and focus on the sensations of touch, gradually rebuilding confidence and trust in their bodies.

2. Cognitive Behavioral Therapy (CBT)

Cognitive Behavioral Therapy (CBT) is a form of psychotherapy that helps men address negative thought patterns that contribute to ED, such as performance anxiety, fear of failure, or self-doubt. CBT focuses on identifying and challenging these thoughts, replacing them with healthier, more constructive beliefs.

<u>Challenging Negative Beliefs</u>: For example, if a man believes that he must always perform perfectly during sex, CBT helps him understand that this expectation is unrealistic and can lead to unnecessary pressure. Instead, he can learn to approach sex with a mindset of exploration, play, and connection.

<u>Reducing Catastrophic Thinking</u>: CBT also helps men reframe their thoughts around ED. Instead of thinking, "If I can't maintain an erection, I'll lose my partner," CBT encourages men to recognize that occasional performance issues are normal and don't necessarily have long-term consequences.

3. Lifestyle Changes That Improve ED

One of the most effective ways to improve erectile function is through lifestyle adjustments. Even small changes can lead to significant improvements in sexual performance.

Exercise Regularly: Cardiovascular exercise improves blood flow, which is critical for erectile function. Activities like running, cycling, and swimming strengthen the heart and promote better circulation. Aim for at least 30 minutes of moderate exercise five times a week.

Eat a Healthy Diet: A diet rich in fruits, vegetables, whole grains, and lean proteins supports overall health, including sexual health. Foods high in antioxidants, like berries and leafy greens, improve blood flow, while reducing processed foods and sugars can help regulate hormone levels.

Reduce Alcohol and Quit Smoking: Excessive drinking and smoking are major contributors to ED. Reducing alcohol consumption and quitting smoking can restore blood vessel health and improve erectile function.

Exercise 3: Building a Healthy Routine

Set Simple Fitness Goals: Choose one or two physical activities you enjoy and commit to doing them consistently. Track your progress each week and note how your body feels during sex or arousal as your fitness improves.

Upgrade Your Diet Gradually: Don't overhaul your diet overnight. Instead, start with small changes, like incorporating more greens into your meals or cutting back on processed snacks. Over time, these adjustments will have a positive impact on your sexual health.

Cut Down on Alcohol: Try reducing alcohol intake by one drink at a time. Set limits before social events or opt for non-alcoholic alternatives. Keeping alcohol consumption in check can prevent it from interfering with sexual performance.

4. Improving Communication and Emotional Connection

For many men, the pressure to perform is heightened by the fear of disappointing their partner. Open, honest communication about sexual expectations, desires, and concerns can relieve this pressure and create a healthier sexual dynamic.

Discussing Fears and Desires: Having regular conversations with your partner about your sexual experiences and desires can help build trust and intimacy. When men feel supported and understood, they are more likely to feel relaxed and confident during sex.

Focusing on Intimacy Beyond Penetration: It's important to remember that intimacy isn't solely defined by penetrative sex. Exploring other forms of physical and emotional connection—such as kissing, cuddling, or oral sex—can reduce performance anxiety and deepen the emotional bond between partners.

Exercise 4: Incorporating Mindfulness Into Sex

Focus on Sensation: During sexual activity, instead of worrying about performance, focus on the physical sensations you're experiencing. Pay attention to your partner's touch, the warmth of their skin, or the rhythm of your breath.

Stop and Breathe: If you feel performance anxiety creeping in, pause for a moment. Take a few deep breaths to calm your mind, and then re-engage in a way that feels natural and pleasurable rather than pressured.

A Holistic Approach to Managing ED

Erectile dysfunction is a common issue that affects men of all ages. By breaking the silence, acknowledging the rise of ED in younger men, and exploring non-medical solutions, you can take control of your sexual health. Lifestyle changes, mindfulness, and open communication with your partner are powerful tools for improving erectile function and overcoming performance anxiety. Remember, ED is not a reflection of your masculinity or your worth—it's a physical and psychological condition that can be addressed with patience, understanding, and proactive steps.

Adopting a holistic approach means focusing not just on the physical aspects of ED but also on mental health, emotional intimacy, and overall well-being. By making small changes to your lifestyle, such as improving your diet, exercising regularly, and managing stress, you can support your body's natural ability to function properly. Additionally, mindfulness practices help you stay grounded during sexual experiences, reducing performance anxiety and improving your overall sexual confidence.

Most importantly, communication is key. Talking openly with your partner about ED fosters trust and eliminates the pressure to perform. Working together as a team can transform what might seem like a challenge into an opportunity to strengthen your physical and emotional relationships.

Erectile dysfunction doesn't define you—it's a manageable condition. With the right tools, mindset, and support, you can regain control of your sexual health and enjoy fulfilling, confident sexual experiences.

Chapter 5: Premature Ejaculation

Premature ejaculation (PE) is one of the most common sexual issues men face, affecting an estimated 30-40% of men at some point in their lives. Yet, despite its prevalence, it is often shrouded in silence and shame. Many men who struggle with PE feel isolated, embarrassed, and anxious about their sexual performance, which only worsens the problem. This chapter seeks to demystify premature ejaculation, explore its causes, examine the emotional toll it can take, and provide practical, shame-free strategies to regain control and confidence in your sex life.

Understanding PE: Why Premature Ejaculation Happens and Its Emotional Toll

What Is Premature Ejaculation?

Premature ejaculation is typically defined as ejaculation that occurs sooner than desired during sexual activity. While there's no universal benchmark for what constitutes "too soon," PE often happens within one to two minutes of penetration and may even occur before penetration begins. It is important to note that the timing of ejaculation is subjective and can vary depending on the individual and the situation. What matters is whether PE causes distress or dissatisfaction for the individual or their partner.

PE can occur occasionally or regularly, and it can be influenced by both physical and psychological factors. There are two primary types of PE:

<u>Primary PE (Lifelong):</u> Men with primary PE have experienced rapid ejaculation since their first sexual experiences. This form of PE is often linked to psychological factors such as anxiety, heightened sensitivity, or learned patterns from early sexual activity.

<u>Secondary PE (Acquired):</u> Secondary PE develops later in life after previously normal sexual performance. This type of PE may be caused by physical conditions such as erectile dysfunction, hormonal imbalances, or psychological issues such as stress, anxiety, or relationship problems.

Why Does Premature Ejaculation Happen?

Premature ejaculation is rarely caused by a single factor. Instead, it's typically the result of a combination of physiological, psychological, and relational influences. Understanding the root causes can help demystify why PE occurs and offer insights into how to address it effectively.

1. Psychological Factors

Performance Anxiety: One of the leading causes of PE is performance anxiety, which creates a cycle of stress and hyper-awareness during sexual activity. When men feel pressured to "perform" and satisfy their partner, this anxiety can heighten arousal to the point where they lose control over ejaculation. The more they focus on avoiding PE, the more likely it is to occur, perpetuating the cycle.

Guilt and Shame: Men who struggle with PE often feel guilty for not meeting their own expectations or their partner's. This guilt can make it difficult to relax during sex, further compounding the problem. Shame around PE can prevent open communication with a partner, leading to feelings of isolation.

Early Sexual Experiences: For men with lifelong PE, early sexual experiences can play a significant role. Men who learned to climax quickly during early encounters—either due to nervousness, inexperience, or a rushed environment—may have developed patterns that persist into adulthood. These learned behaviors are difficult to unlearn without conscious effort.

Depression and Emotional Stress: Depression and emotional stress can also contribute to PE. Depression often affects libido and sexual performance, while emotional stress related to work, family, or relationships can disrupt focus and arousal during sex.

2. Biological Factors

Hormonal Imbalances: Low serotonin levels, a neurotransmitter that helps regulate mood and sexual function, are thought to be linked to PE. Serotonin plays a role in delaying ejaculation, and an imbalance can lead to quicker arousal and less control.

Erectile Dysfunction (ED): Men with erectile dysfunction sometimes experience PE as they may rush to climax before losing their erection. This secondary PE is common in men with ED, and addressing the underlying erectile issues can help alleviate PE.

Hypersensitivity: Some men may have a heightened sensitivity of the penis, which makes it more difficult to delay ejaculation. Hypersensitivity can be physical (due to nerve endings) or psychological (linked to heightened arousal).

Genetic Factors: There is evidence to suggest that PE may have a genetic component, with some men being more predisposed to rapid ejaculation due to inherited biological traits.

The Emotional Toll of Premature Ejaculation

Premature ejaculation doesn't just affect a man's sexual performance—it can take a serious emotional toll as well. Men who struggle with PE may experience feelings of shame, guilt, frustration, and inadequacy. Over time, these emotions can erode self-confidence and create anxiety around sexual encounters, further perpetuating the problem.

1. Impact on Self-Esteem and Masculinity

For many men, sexual performance is deeply tied to their sense of masculinity and self-worth. When PE interferes with their ability to satisfy a partner or live up to their own expectations, it can lead to feelings of inadequacy. Men may start to question their value as lovers and, by extension, as men. This can create a cycle of negative self-talk and self-blame, which erodes confidence in and out of the bedroom.

2. Impact on Relationships

PE can also have a significant impact on relationships. Men may avoid initiating sex out of fear of disappointing their partner, which can lead to emotional and physical distance. Partners may feel unsatisfied or frustrated, though they may be reluctant to express these feelings for fear of hurting their partner's ego. This lack of communication can breed resentment on both sides, further damaging intimacy.

However, it's important to remember that open communication and mutual understanding are key to overcoming PE. Many partners are understanding and supportive when men are honest about their struggles, and together they can work to find solutions that improve their sexual connection.

3. Anxiety and Avoidance

The fear of "failing" during sex can cause men to develop sexual avoidance behaviors. They may avoid initiating sex, withdraw emotionally, or rely on distractions to avoid facing the issue directly. This only intensifies the emotional burden, creating more anxiety and stress around sex.

Practical, Shame-Free Solutions for Overcoming Premature Ejaculation

Premature ejaculation is a treatable issue, and overcoming it requires a combination of physical techniques, psychological approaches, and open communication with a partner. The goal is to reduce performance pressure, increase awareness of sexual sensations, and develop better control over ejaculation—all without shame or judgment.

1. Mindfulness and Sensate Focus Techniques

Mindfulness techniques can help men focus on the present moment, reducing anxiety and heightening body awareness. By practicing mindfulness during sex, men can shift their attention away from performance goals and focus on the sensations and connection with their partner.

How It Works:

Breathing Control: As you begin sexual activity, focus on slow, deep breathing. When you feel your arousal rising quickly, pause and take several deep breaths to calm your body.

Focus on Sensations: Instead of rushing toward orgasm, focus on the entire experience—your partner's touch, the warmth of their skin, the rhythm of your breathing. This slows the pace and helps you maintain control.

2. The Start-Stop Technique: Regaining Control

The "stop-start" method is one of the most widely recommended techniques for managing PE. This approach involves stimulating the penis until the man feels he's about to ejaculate, then stopping all stimulation until the sensation subsides. By practicing this technique during masturbation or with a partner, men can gradually learn to delay ejaculation and increase their control.

How It Works:

Begin Stimulation: Engage in sexual activity or masturbation and focus on the sensations in your body.

Pause Before Orgasm: As you feel yourself approaching ejaculation, stop all stimulation and focus on relaxing your body. You'll notice the urge to ejaculate diminishes as your arousal levels decrease.

Resume: Once you feel back in control, resume stimulation and repeat the process. Over time, you'll gain better control over your arousal and ejaculatory response.

Exercise 1: Practicing the Start-Stop Technique Alone
Solo Practice: Start by using this technique during masturbation. Pay attention to your body's signals as you reach the point of no return and train yourself to pause before reaching orgasm.

Track Your Progress: Each time you practice, try to extend the time it takes to reach ejaculation by a few seconds. As you improve, you'll notice a greater sense of control during partnered sex as well.

3. The Squeeze Technique: Physical Control

Similar to the stop-start method, the squeeze technique involves applying pressure to the penis just before ejaculation to reduce arousal and delay climax. Typically, a man (or his partner) applies pressure to the area just below the head of the penis for several seconds until the urge to ejaculate decreases. Afterward, stimulation can resume. With regular practice, this technique helps increase ejaculatory control.

How It Works:

<u>Squeeze the Base</u>: When you feel the urge to ejaculate, firmly but gently squeeze the base of the penis (or have your partner do so). This temporarily reduces arousal and delays ejaculation.

<u>Wait and Resume</u>: After the squeeze, pause for a few moments before resuming stimulation. Over time, this can help train your body to delay ejaculation naturally.

Exercise 2: Squeeze Technique with a Partner

<u>Communicate with Your Partner</u>: Explain to your partner that you'd like to try the squeeze technique together to increase control. Let them know when you feel close to climax, and have them assist by applying gentle pressure to the base of the penis.

Practice Together: Incorporating this into your sexual routine can help strengthen the bond with your partner and make the process more collaborative and fun.

Exercise 3: Mindfulness Practice for Sexual Control

Pre-Sex Mindfulness: Spend 5-10 minutes before sexual activity practicing mindfulness. Sit quietly, close your eyes, and focus on your breath. Inhale for 4 counts, hold for 4, and exhale for 6. This will help you stay calm and in control when you begin sexual activity.

Mindful Touching: During sex, engage in mindful touching with your partner—explore each other's bodies without rushing toward intercourse. This allows you to stay grounded in the experience rather than focusing on the outcome.

4. Strengthening the Pelvic Floor Muscles

Kegel exercises, which involve contracting and relaxing the pelvic floor muscles, can improve ejaculatory control by strengthening the muscles responsible for ejaculation. These exercises can be done daily and are discreet, making them an easy addition to any routine.

How It Works:

Kegel Exercises: Kegels involve contracting and relaxing the pelvic floor muscles (the same muscles you use to stop the flow of urine).

Identify the Muscle: Next time you urinate, stop mid-flow. The muscles you engage are your pelvic floor muscles.

Exercise: Contract those muscles, hold for 5 seconds, and then relax for 5 seconds. Repeat this 10-15 times, three times a day. Stronger pelvic floor muscles give you better control over ejaculation.

5. Cognitive Behavioral Therapy (CBT)

Cognitive Behavioral Therapy (CBT) can help men address the psychological factors contributing to PE, such as performance anxiety, negative self-talk, or unhelpful beliefs about sex. CBT focuses on reframing negative thought patterns and creating healthier, more constructive beliefs about sexual performance.

Reframing Negative Thoughts: For example, instead of thinking, "I'll never satisfy my partner," CBT encourages men to recognize that sexual satisfaction comes from connection, not just performance. Reframing these beliefs can reduce anxiety and build confidence over time.

Shame-Free Solutions: Approaching PE with Confidence

Premature ejaculation can carry a lot of shame, but it's important to understand that it's a common issue and doesn't define your worth or masculinity. The key is to approach PE with confidence and openness, both with yourself and your partner.

1. Open Communication with Your Partner

One of the most important aspects of overcoming PE is talking openly with your partner about what's happening. Many men avoid discussing PE out of fear of disappointing their partner, but most partners appreciate honesty and want to help. By discussing the issue, you can work together to find solutions that reduce pressure and create a more supportive, understanding sexual dynamic.

<u>Focus on Connection</u>: Remember that sex is about more than penetration and climax—it's about intimacy, connection, and shared pleasure. By focusing on these aspects, both partners can feel fulfilled, even if PE occurs.

<u>Be Honest</u>: If PE is affecting your sexual experiences, talk to your partner. Explain that this is something you're working on and express your desire to make sex fulfilling for both of you. Opening up reduces the tension and can foster more cooperation in finding solutions.

<u>Reframe the Experience</u>: Instead of viewing PE as a failure, reframe it as an opportunity to explore other forms of intimacy—prolonged foreplay, non-penetrative sex, or playful exploration of each other's bodies. Focus on the pleasure and connection rather than the performance.

Exercise 4: The Intimacy Conversation

Initiate a Conversation: Find a relaxed time to talk with your partner. Start with a positive approach: "I really value our connection, and I'd like to talk about ways we can make our sex life even more enjoyable for both of us."

Express Your Intentions: Share that you've been working on techniques to improve control and that you'd love their support in the process. This helps bring your partner into the experience as a collaborator rather than placing all the pressure on yourself.

2. Cultivating Self-Compassion

The biggest hurdle in dealing with PE is often internal. Men tend to be hard on themselves, equating premature ejaculation with failure. Learning to treat yourself with compassion is critical to overcoming the shame.

Practice Self-Forgiveness: Understand that PE is a common issue, not a personal failing. If you experience PE, remind yourself that it's part of the process of learning and improving.

Focus on Progress, Not Perfection: The goal is not to be perfect but to improve control over time. Celebrate small wins, like lasting a little longer or feeling more connected to your partner during sex.

Exercise 5: Self-Compassion Journaling

Reflect on Your Progress: After each sexual experience, write down one thing that went well—lasting longer, communicating openly, or simply enjoying the connection with your partner.

Write a Compassionate Letter to Yourself: If you experience frustration or shame, take a moment to write a letter to yourself as though you were comforting a friend. Remind yourself that PE doesn't define you and that improvement takes time.

Approaching PE with Confidence and Control

Premature ejaculation is a common and treatable issue. By
addressing the underlying causes—either psychological,
emotional, or physical—men can regain control over their
sexual performance and rebuild their confidence in the
bedroom. The key to overcoming PE is approaching the
problem with patience, self-compassion, and a willingness
to experiment with different techniques.

PE does not define you as a man, and it doesn't have to
dictate the quality of your sexual relationships. With the
right tools, open communication, and a focus on emotional
and physical connection, you can regain control and
experience a fulfilling, confident sex life.

☐

Chapter 6: Porn-Induced Sexual Issues

In today's digital age, pornography is more accessible than ever before. With just a few clicks, men can find themselves immersed in an endless stream of sexual content that can range from the mundane to the extreme. While watching porn occasionally is not inherently harmful, for many men, heavy consumption of pornography has a significant impact on their sexual health, relationships, and performance. This chapter explores the complex relationship between pornography and real sex and how porn consumption can distort expectations and performance. It provides practical steps for recognizing and addressing porn-induced sexual issues, including porn addiction. Finally, we will offer actionable strategies to help men rewire their brains and reconnect with genuine intimacy and pleasure in their sexual relationships.

Porn and Its Impact on Real Sex

Understanding the Disconnect Between Porn and Real Sex

Pornography often portrays highly stylized, exaggerated, and unrealistic depictions of sex. While it may seem like harmless entertainment, consuming large amounts of porn can warp men's expectations of what sex should be like, both physically and emotionally. This disconnect can lead to frustration, dissatisfaction, and even performance issues in real-life sexual encounters.

1. Unrealistic Portrayals of Bodies and Performance

Pornographic films often showcase performers with idealized bodies—men who are exceptionally muscular and well-endowed and women who are perfectly proportioned with flawless skin. In addition to their physical attributes, porn performers engage in exaggerated sexual activities that are often void of emotional connection. These depictions create an unrealistic standard for how men believe their bodies should look and how sex should unfold.

<u>Physical Expectations</u>: Men may begin to believe that they need to look a certain way or have a certain penis size to be sexually attractive or capable of satisfying a partner. This can lead to body image issues and performance anxiety when reality does not align with the images they've consumed.

<u>Endurance and Performance Pressure</u>: In many porn scenes, male performers engage in marathon-length sexual acts, often lasting for what seems like hours. In reality, the average sexual encounter is much shorter, and many of these scenes are edited or involve breaks to maintain the illusion of endurance. Men who consume large amounts of porn may develop unrealistic expectations about how long they should last or how they should perform, leading to anxiety and disappointment when their real-life sexual experiences do not match.

2. The Absence of Emotional Connection

One of the most significant differences between porn and real-life sex is the lack of emotional intimacy portrayed in pornography. In most mainstream pornographic content, the focus is purely on physical pleasure and sexual acts, with little regard for emotional connection, communication, or consent. Real-life sex, however, involves a complex interplay of emotions, intimacy, and mutual understanding between partners.

<u>Emotional Detachment</u>: For men who consume large amounts of porn, there is often a detachment from the emotional aspects of sex. They may become more focused on physical pleasure and visual stimulation rather than the emotional connection from engaging with a partner. This can lead to difficulties in achieving emotional satisfaction during real-life sexual experiences, leaving both partners feeling unfulfilled.

The Impact of Heavy Porn Consumption on Sexual Health

While occasional porn consumption is unlikely to cause harm, heavy or habitual use of pornography can have a profound effect on sexual health, performance, and relationships. The brain's reward system, which is responsible for processing pleasure and reinforcing behaviors, is highly sensitive to stimuli like pornography. Over time, excessive consumption of porn can rewire the brain, leading to a range of sexual performance issues and emotional disconnects.

1. Porn-Induced Erectile Dysfunction (PIED)

One of the most common issues men experience as a result
of heavy porn use is porn-induced erectile dysfunction
(PIED). Unlike traditional erectile dysfunction, which is
often caused by physical health issues, PIED occurs when
men become so accustomed to the hyper-stimulation of porn
that they struggle to become aroused or maintain an
erection during real-life sexual encounters.

<u>Desensitization to Real Sex</u>: Porn provides instant
gratification, offering novelty and extreme visual stimuli
that flood the brain with dopamine—the neurotransmitter
responsible for pleasure. Over time, the brain becomes
desensitized to these dopamine surges, requiring more
extreme or novel content to achieve the same level of
arousal. This can make it difficult for men to become
aroused by real-life sexual situations, where the sensory
input is more subtle and emotionally nuanced.

<u>Decreased Arousal During Partnered Sex</u>: Many men with
PIED report that while they can easily become aroused by
pornography, they struggle to maintain erections or
experience sexual excitement with their partners. This
leads to frustration, anxiety, and a sense of inadequacy,
which only perpetuates the cycle of erectile dysfunction.

<u>Unrealistic Sexual Scripts</u>: Men may expect their partners
to act like porn stars, leading to dissatisfaction when reality
doesn't match those scripts. This can create tension,
disappointment, and unrealistic pressure on both partners.

2. Increased Performance Anxiety

Porn-induced performance anxiety is another common issue among men who consume a significant amount of pornography. Men who internalize the exaggerated performances they see in porn may develop unrealistic expectations about their own sexual abilities. This can lead to anxiety about their ability to perform in bed, particularly when it comes to stamina, erection strength, or how quickly they reach orgasm.

<u>Fear of Not Measuring Up</u>: Men who are accustomed to seeing porn actors perform for extended periods, with exaggerated expressions of pleasure from their partners, may fear that they do not measure up in their sexual encounters. This can create a sense of inadequacy and pressure, making it difficult to relax and enjoy sex.

<u>Avoidance of Real-Life Sex</u>: For some men, the fear of underperforming or not being able to satisfy their partner becomes so overwhelming that they avoid sexual encounters altogether. This avoidance can create tension in relationships, increase feelings of isolation, and exacerbate sexual performance issues.

3. Emotional Detachment and Relationship Issues

In addition to performance issues, heavy porn consumption can lead to emotional detachment and problems in relationships. Men who use pornography as their primary source of sexual stimulation may find it difficult to connect emotionally with their partners, leading to feelings of distance, dissatisfaction, and even resentment from both parties.

Objectification of Partners: Pornography often reduces sex to a purely physical act, devoid of emotional intimacy or connection. Over time, this can lead men to view their partners as objects of pleasure rather than equals in a mutually fulfilling relationship. This objectification can cause men to miss out on the deeper emotional aspects of sex, leading to dissatisfaction and frustration in their relationships.

Erosion of Trust and Communication: If a partner feels neglected or disconnected because of heavy porn use, trust can be eroded. Open communication is essential in maintaining a healthy sexual relationship, and hiding or lying about porn consumption can create emotional distance and resentment.

Exercise 1: Identifying the Impact of Porn on Your Sex Life

Reflect on Your Usage: Write down how often you use porn and if it has impacted your sexual satisfaction. Do you notice a difference in your desire for real sex versus porn? Are you less aroused or excited by real-life sexual encounters?

Compare Expectations to Reality: List some expectations you have about sex (e.g., duration, body appearance, intensity) and compare them to your real-life experiences. Are your expectations realistic? What aspects of real sex do you enjoy that porn doesn't show?

Evaluate Emotional Connection: Reflect on your emotional connection during sex with a partner. Do you find it harder to stay emotionally present or connected? How does your porn usage impact your ability to experience pleasure with a partner?

Porn Addiction: Recognizing When Porn Use Becomes Problematic

What Is Porn Addiction?

For some men, pornography consumption goes beyond occasional use and becomes a compulsive behavior. Porn addiction, much like other forms of addiction, involves the inability to control consumption, despite negative consequences in one's life, relationships, or mental health. Recognizing the signs of porn addiction is the first step in addressing the problem.

Signs of Porn Addiction:

Escalation of Consumption: A need to watch increasingly extreme or novel pornography to achieve the same level of arousal.

Inability to Stop: Despite wanting to cut back or stop watching porn, you find it difficult or impossible to do so.

Neglecting Responsibilities: Spending excessive amounts of time watching porn, to the point where it interferes with work, social obligations, or relationships.

Negative Emotional Impact: Feeling guilt, shame, or depression related to your porn use but continuing to engage in the behavior.

Loss of Interest in Real Sex: Preferring porn to real-life sexual encounters with a partner or finding it difficult to become aroused by real sex.

The Emotional and Psychological Effects of Porn Addiction

Porn addiction can take a toll on mental health, leading to feelings of guilt, shame, anxiety, or depression. The constant need to seek sexual gratification through porn can create a sense of isolation and emotional disconnection from partners, family, and friends.

Porn addiction can also lead to:

Performance Anxiety: The fear of not being able to perform sexually without porn-induced arousal.

Body Dysmorphia: Constant comparison to porn actors can lead to feelings of inadequacy regarding body size, genital appearance, or stamina.

Relationship Strain: Porn addiction can create distrust or distance in relationships, especially if it's hidden or if a partner feels neglected in favor of pornography.

Exercise 2: Assessing Your Relationship with Porn

Track Your Usage: For one week, track how often you watch porn and the circumstances around it. Are you using it out of habit, boredom, or stress? This helps identify patterns of compulsive behavior.

Evaluate Consequences: Reflect on if your porn consumption has had negative effects on your life, such as decreased interest in sex, relationship issues, or feelings of guilt or shame. Write down these consequences and consider how they've impacted your well-being.

Seek Professional Help: If you recognize signs of addiction, consider speaking to a therapist or counselor who specializes in sexual health or addiction. Therapy can provide tools to address underlying issues and develop healthier coping mechanisms.

Rewiring Your Brain for Real Sex

Porn addiction and over-reliance on pornography can be addressed through a conscious effort to rewire the brain for genuine intimacy. This involves reducing porn consumption, reconnecting with your body, and rediscovering pleasure in real-life sexual experiences.

1. Taking a Break: Porn Detox

The first step in overcoming porn-induced sexual issues is to take a break from pornography. This break gives your brain time to reset its reward system and reduce the desensitization caused by excessive dopamine release. During this time, you may experience cravings or urges to return to porn, but it's important to resist these impulses and focus on healthier forms of sexual stimulation.

How to Start a Porn Detox:

<u>Set a Goal</u>: Commit to a specific period (e.g., 30 days) where you abstain from watching porn. This gives your brain time to recalibrate.

<u>Replace the Habit</u>: Instead of watching porn, engage in other activities that bring you pleasure or relaxation, such as exercise, reading, or spending quality time with your partner.

<u>Journal Your Experience</u>: Keep a journal during your detox to track how you're feeling—both physically and emotionally. This will help you stay mindful of the benefits of reducing porn use.

2. Rediscovering Real-Life Intimacy

Restoring emotional intimacy is a critical part of overcoming porn-induced sexual issues. By focusing on emotional connection rather than physical performance, you can create a more satisfying and fulfilling sexual relationship with your partner.

<u>Focus on Emotional Connection</u>: Prioritize emotional closeness and intimacy over physical gratification. Spend time talking, cuddling, or engaging in non-sexual activities that strengthen your bond with your partner.

<u>Explore New Forms of Pleasure</u>: Instead of focusing solely on penetration or orgasm, explore other forms of sexual

pleasure, like sensual touch, massage, or extended foreplay. This helps shift your focus away from the porn-induced "script" and toward mutual enjoyment.

Practice Mindful Sex: Mindfulness helps you stay present during sex, making it easier to focus on sensations and connection rather than chasing unrealistic porn expectations.

Exercise 3: Reconnecting with Your Partner

Engage in Non-Sexual Intimacy: Spend time with your partner engaging in non-sexual forms of intimacy. Go for a walk, talk about your day, or give each other massages; this helps strengthen your emotional connection and reminds you that intimacy isn't solely about sex.

Introduce Mindfulness: During sexual activity, focus on being fully present. Pay attention to your breathing, your partner's touch, and the sensations in your body. This helps rewire your brain to appreciate real-life physical connection over artificial stimulation.

3. Engage in Mindfulness and Sensory Awareness

Mindfulness practices can help you become more aware of your body, sensations, and emotions during sexual experiences. By focusing on the present moment and paying attention to how your body feels, you can increase your sensitivity to real-life sexual stimuli and reduce the need for hyper-stimulation provided by pornography.

Mindful Masturbation: If you choose to masturbate, do so without the aid of pornography or visual stimuli. Focus on how your body feels, the sensations of touch, and your breath. This practice helps you reconnect with your body and reduces the reliance on visual stimulation for arousal.

Sensate Focus with Your Partner: Sensate focus exercises, which involve exploring non-sexual touch and gradually building to sexual contact, can help you and your partner reconnect physically and emotionally. This practice reduces performance pressure and helps both partners focus on the sensations of touch and pleasure rather than the goal of orgasm.

4. Physical and Mental Health Practices

Addressing porn addiction also requires attention to your overall well-being. Improving your physical and mental health can make it easier to break the habit and enjoy more fulfilling sexual experiences.

Exercise: Regular exercise improves circulation, increases energy, and reduces stress—all of which contribute to better sexual performance and satisfaction.

Therapy or Counseling: If porn use is rooted in deeper emotional or psychological issues (such as loneliness, anxiety, or unresolved trauma), therapy can help you work through those challenges.

Exercise 4: Building a New Routine
Create a Daily Routine Without Porn: Replace your usual porn-watching habits with activities that support your well-being. This could include physical exercise, practicing mindfulness, or spending time doing hobbies you enjoy.

Focus on Self-Care: Take care of your body and mind through healthy eating, sleep, and stress-reducing activities. The better you feel physically and mentally, the easier it will be to reduce the reliance on porn for gratification.

5. Cognitive Behavioral Therapy (CBT)

For men who struggle with compulsive porn use or porn-induced performance issues, cognitive behavioral therapy (CBT) can be a valuable tool. CBT helps individuals identify and change negative thought patterns and behaviors, replacing them with healthier coping mechanisms.

Reframing Negative Beliefs: For example, if you believe that you need porn to become aroused, CBT helps you challenge that belief by focusing on other sources of pleasure, such as emotional intimacy or physical touch.

Addressing Performance Anxiety: CBT can also help reduce performance anxiety by challenging unrealistic expectations about sex. Instead of focusing on perfect performance, you can learn to focus on connection, communication, and shared pleasure with your partner.

Reclaiming Intimacy and Reducing Porn Reliance

Porn-induced sexual issues can be challenging to overcome, but they aren't insurmountable. By recognizing the impact of pornography on your sexual expectations and performance, addressing addiction, and rewiring your brain for real sex, you can rediscover intimacy and satisfaction. The conclusion is that reclaiming genuine intimacy is not about cutting out pleasure but about rediscovering how to enjoy it in healthy, real-life contexts. As you reduce reliance on porn, reconnect with your partner, and engage in mindful practices, you'll begin to see improvements in your sexual confidence and performance. This journey requires patience, but the rewards—deeper emotional connection, more fulfilling sex, and improved self-esteem—are well worth the effort.

PART III: The Emotional and Psychological Side of Sex

Sexuality is closely connected to emotional and psychological health, and the way men handle these dimensions of their sexual lives can significantly affect their overall well-being and relationship satisfaction. While the physical side of sex often takes center stage, the emotional and mental aspects are equally important. In this section, we will delve into the emotional and psychological factors that shape men's sexual experiences—from anxiety and self-esteem challenges to the role of emotional intimacy and openness.

By addressing these emotional and psychological challenges, men can develop a more holistic understanding of their sexual lives, build deeper connections with their partners, and foster greater self-awareness and confidence.

Chapter 7: Emotional Intimacy and Vulnerability

Unlocking Deeper Connections

Emotional intimacy is the cornerstone of any healthy and fulfilling relationship, but for many men, expressing emotions openly, especially in the context of sex, can feel challenging or even impossible. From a young age, cultural conditioning often teaches men to separate emotion from sexual experiences, emphasizing physical performance and dominance over emotional connection. This distancing can prevent men from establishing the deep emotional bonds that are essential for long-term relationship satisfaction. In this chapter, we'll explore why men struggle with emotional openness, how vulnerability can be a source of strength and the importance of communicating emotional and sexual needs to create more meaningful connections.

For many men, emotional openness feels like stepping into uncharted territory. Society often dictates that men should be tough, stoic, and in control at all times, viewing vulnerability as a sign of weakness. These messages, reinforced throughout a man's life, create barriers that make it difficult to express emotions—especially in relationships and sexual contexts.

1. Cultural Conditioning and Gender Roles

From an early age, many boys are taught that emotions like sadness, fear, or insecurity are feminine traits and therefore should be suppressed. They are often encouraged to "man up," "toughen up," or "stop crying," leading to a belief that expressing emotions makes them appear weak or unmanly. Instead, they are rewarded for stoicism, independence, and physical strength. Over time, this conditioning teaches men that they should avoid discussing or acknowledging their emotions, particularly in intimate relationships.

<u>Emotional Avoidance</u>: As a result of this conditioning, many men avoid discussing their emotions or bury them under layers of humor, detachment, or aggression. In the context of sex, this avoidance can lead to a focus on performance and physical pleasure rather than emotional connection and intimacy.

<u>Fear of Vulnerability</u>: Because society often equates vulnerability with weakness, many men develop a fear of being emotionally exposed. They may worry that opening up about their emotions will make them seem inadequate, unworthy, or less masculine in the eyes of their partner. This fear of vulnerability prevents men from engaging in the deep emotional exchanges that can strengthen relationships.

2. The Pressure to Perform

In the context of sex, the pressure to perform can be a significant barrier to emotional intimacy. Many men view sex as an area where they must excel and prove their worth as lovers. This performance-based mindset focuses on physical acts—erection, stamina, and orgasm—rather than emotional connection. When men feel pressured to meet certain physical standards, they may become disconnected from their emotions, focusing solely on "doing it right" rather than being fully present with their partner.

<u>The Disconnect Between Performance and Connection</u>: Men who focus solely on sexual performance may neglect the emotional aspects of sex, such as feeling connected, loved, or appreciated by their partner. This can lead to a shallow sexual experience that leaves both partners feeling unfulfilled, even if the sex itself is physically satisfying.

3. Emotional Inexperience

For many men, emotional inexperience can make vulnerability and emotional intimacy feel unfamiliar or uncomfortable. If a man has never been encouraged to explore or express his feelings, he may not have the tools to communicate his emotions effectively. This lack of experience can lead to discomfort or anxiety when trying to open up in intimate situations, leaving men unsure of how to navigate the emotional side of relationships.

<u>Emotional Numbness</u>: Emotional inexperience can result in numbness or detachment from feelings. Men may struggle to recognize or articulate their emotions, making it harder to engage in meaningful conversations with their partners about their needs and desires.

The Impact on Relationships

When men are emotionally disconnected during sex, it can leave their partners feeling distant or unimportant. Emotional openness fosters trust and a sense of being seen and understood. Without it, relationships can struggle, with one partner feeling emotionally neglected while the other feels the pressure to meet unrealistic performance standards.

Key Consequences Include:

<u>Increased Performance Anxiety</u>: Focusing solely on the physical aspects of sex can heighten performance anxiety, making it harder to enjoy the experience.

<u>Emotional Disconnection</u>: Without emotional intimacy, sex may feel mechanical or unfulfilling for both partners.

<u>Unresolved Needs</u>: When men avoid discussing their emotional and sexual needs, it leaves gaps in the relationship that can lead to frustration and resentment.

Emotional Vulnerability as Strength

Reframing Vulnerability

The idea that emotional vulnerability is a weakness is outdated and untrue. In reality, emotional vulnerability is a powerful strength that can deepen relationships and foster a stronger sense of connection. By opening up emotionally, men allow themselves to be seen for who they truly are, building trust with their partners and creating space for deeper intimacy.

In the context of sex, emotional vulnerability means sharing not just your physical desires but also your emotional experiences—your fears, insecurities, desires for connection, and what sex means to you beyond the physical act. This openness can transform sex from a purely physical experience to one that is emotionally and spiritually fulfilling for both partners.

1. The Power of Emotional Honesty

Emotional honesty is about being real with yourself and your partner. It involves acknowledging and expressing your true feelings, even when they're difficult or uncomfortable. Being emotionally honest requires vulnerability because it means putting aside the fear of being judged or misunderstood and showing up as your authentic self.

<u>Building Trust Through Openness</u>: When men are emotionally honest, they invite their partner to do the same. This creates a space of mutual trust and respect where both partners feel safe sharing their thoughts and feelings. Emotional honesty can deepen the connection between partners and foster a greater sense of intimacy inside and outside the bedroom.

<u>Reducing Anxiety and Shame</u>: Keeping emotions bottled up can lead to anxiety and shame, especially in the context of sexual performance. By being open about feelings of insecurity, fear, or doubt, men can relieve some of the pressure they place on themselves. This emotional release

can lead to a more relaxed and satisfying sexual experience, free from the fear of judgment or failure.

2. Vulnerability Enhances Sexual Connection

When men are willing to be vulnerable, they create the opportunity for a more connected and fulfilling sexual experience. Sex is not just about physical pleasure; it's about emotional intimacy and mutual connection. By sharing their emotions with their partner, men can deepen the emotional bond and create a stronger sense of trust and closeness during sex.

<u>Fostering Emotional Intimacy During Sex</u>: Emotional intimacy enhances sexual pleasure by creating a deeper connection between partners. When both partners feel emotionally secure and open, they can fully engage in the sexual experience without the distractions of performance anxiety or emotional detachment. This emotional connection often leads to more fulfilling and satisfying sex, as both partners feel understood and valued.

<u>Communicating Needs and Desires</u>: Vulnerability also allows men to express their sexual needs and desires more openly. Many men struggle to communicate what they truly want in bed, either because they fear being judged or because they've been conditioned to put their partner's needs first. By embracing vulnerability, men can have honest conversations about their desires, preferences, and boundaries, leading to a more satisfying sexual relationship for both partners.

Stronger Bond with Your Partner: Emotional vulnerability creates a sense of closeness and trust, making both partners feel more secure and connected.

Increased Sexual Satisfaction: When you are emotionally open, sex becomes more about mutual pleasure and connection rather than performance. This leads to more fulfilling and enjoyable sexual experiences.

Reduced Performance Anxiety: Vulnerability helps take the pressure off performance by shifting the focus to emotional connection and pleasure.

Exercise 1: Practicing Emotional Vulnerability in Small Steps

Start with Non-Sexual Intimacy: Before focusing on emotional openness during sex, start by sharing your feelings outside the bedroom. For example, tell your partner about a recent challenge you faced at work or something that made you feel vulnerable emotionally.

Share an Emotional Experience During Sex: During intimate moments, try sharing what you're feeling emotionally. It could be as simple as, "I feel really close to you right now," or "I love how connected we are." This can help create a more emotionally intimate atmosphere.

Focus on Your Partner's Emotions: Ask your partner how they're feeling emotionally during or after sex. This opens the door to mutual emotional expression and deepens the connection.

Communicating Your Needs

Why Men Avoid Sharing Emotional and Sexual Needs

Many men avoid sharing their emotional and sexual needs out of fear of judgment, rejection, or appearing weak. They may worry that expressing these needs will make them seem less masculine or too demanding. However, not communicating these needs can lead to frustration, dissatisfaction, and a sense of disconnection in the relationship.

The Importance of Clear Communication

Communication is key in any healthy relationship. Learning to express your emotional and sexual needs not only improves intimacy but also helps both partners feel more satisfied and understood. By opening up, you create space for your partner to understand what you need to feel connected, respected, and loved.

When communication about needs is avoided, assumptions and misunderstandings arise, creating distance between partners. Clear communication, on the other hand, fosters understanding, empathy, and stronger emotional bonds.

• Active Listening: Listening is one of the most powerful tools for emotional intimacy. When men practice active listening—fully focusing on their partner's words without interruption or judgment—they show that they value and respect their partner's emotions. This creates a reciprocal environment where both partners feel heard and understood.

• <u>Non-Judgmental Communication</u>: Men should aim to communicate their emotions without fear of being judged. Sharing feelings like fear, insecurity, or frustration doesn't make a man weak—it makes him human. When partners approach each other with empathy and understanding, they create a deeper emotional bond that strengthens the relationship.

Expressing Sexual Desires and Boundaries

Just as emotional needs must be communicated, so must sexual desires and boundaries. Many men struggle to express what they want sexually, either out of fear of being seen as selfish or because they've been conditioned to prioritize their partner's pleasure over their own.

<u>Honest Conversations About Sex</u>: Men should feel comfortable expressing their sexual desires and preferences in a non-judgmental space. This may include discussing things like sexual fantasies, turn-ons, or specific needs in bed. When men are open about their sexual desires, it fosters a sense of trust and mutual respect between partners.

<u>Respecting Boundaries</u>: Vulnerability isn't just about expressing desires—it's also about being honest when something doesn't feel right. Men should communicate their sexual boundaries and feel empowered to say "no" to

activities that make them uncomfortable. This helps create a safe and respectful sexual environment where both partners' needs are valued.

How to Express Emotional and Sexual Needs

Use "I" Statements: Instead of framing your needs as complaints or criticisms, use "I" statements to express how you feel. For example, instead of saying, "You never initiate sex," try, "I would love it if you initiated sex sometimes. It would make me feel desired and connected."

Be Honest and Direct: While it might feel uncomfortable at first, being honest about your needs is key. Avoid skirting around the issue—be direct but compassionate in your communication.

Focus on Solutions Together: If a need isn't being met, frame the conversation as an opportunity for growth and connection. Say something like, "I've been feeling a bit disconnected lately. How do you feel about finding ways to reconnect emotionally and sexually?"

Exercise 2: Communicating Your Needs

Write Down Your Needs: Before having a conversation with your partner, take some time to write down what your emotional and sexual needs are. Be as specific as possible— do you need more affection? More verbal affirmation? More physical intimacy?

Choose the Right Time: Timing is important when discussing needs. Avoid bringing it up during a heated moment or right after sex. Instead, choose a time when you and your partner are both calm and open to discussion.

Invite a Two-Way Conversation: After expressing your needs, invite your partner to share theirs. Ask questions like, "What do you need from me to feel more connected?" This creates a balanced dialogue where both partners feel heard.

Practical Steps for Cultivating Emotional Intimacy

Cultivating emotional intimacy takes time, patience, and practice. The following strategies can help men overcome their fear of vulnerability and build deeper emotional connections with their partner.

1. Practice Emotional Awareness

Emotional awareness is the ability to recognize and understand your feelings. Many men struggle with emotional awareness because they've been conditioned to ignore or suppress their emotions. By practicing emotional awareness, men can begin to identify their feelings and understand how those emotions affect their relationships.

Journaling: Keeping a journal is a helpful way to practice emotional awareness. By writing down your thoughts and feelings each day, you can gain insight into your emotional state and identify patterns in how you react to different situations.

Mindfulness Meditation: Mindfulness meditation can help men become more in tune with their emotions. By practicing mindfulness, men can learn to observe their feelings without judgment, allowing them to process emotions in a healthy and constructive way.

2. Take Small Steps Toward Vulnerability

If the idea of opening up emotionally feels daunting, start by taking small steps toward vulnerability. You don't have to share everything all at once. Instead, begin by sharing small pieces of your emotional world with your partner and gradually build up your comfort level over time.

Share Something Personal: Start by sharing something personal that you haven't discussed with your partner before. It could be a fear, a dream, or an experience that had a significant impact on you. This helps create a foundation of trust and emotional openness.

Acknowledge Your Emotions in Real-Time: If you feel yourself becoming emotional during a conversation, try to acknowledge it in real-time. For example, you might say, "I'm feeling a bit overwhelmed right now," or "I'm nervous about sharing this, but I want to be honest with you." This shows your partner that you're willing to be vulnerable, even when it's uncomfortable.

3. Encourage Emotional Intimacy in Sexual Relationships

To deepen emotional intimacy during sex, men should focus on the emotional connection with their partner, rather than just the physical aspects of the experience.

<u>Slow Down</u>: Take time to savor the emotional and physical sensations during sex. Slow down, make eye contact, and focus on the emotional connection between you and your partner. This helps build intimacy and creates a more fulfilling sexual experience.

<u>Talk About Sex</u>: After sex, take the time to talk about how the experience felt for both you and your partner. Discuss what you enjoyed, what made you feel connected, and any emotions that came up during the experience. This creates a space for emotional intimacy and reinforces the connection between you and your partner.

Embracing Emotional Intimacy for Deeper Connection

Emotional intimacy is not just a bonus in relationships—it's a foundation for deeper connection, trust, and satisfaction in and out of the bedroom. While many men have been conditioned to separate emotions from sex, learning to communicate needs can transform relationships, making them more fulfilling, supportive, and intimate.

By opening up emotionally, you strengthen the bond with your partner and improve your own emotional well-being. Emotional intimacy is a two-way street, and when both partners feel comfortable sharing their feelings, desires, and needs, the relationship becomes a place of mutual growth and love.

☐

Chapter 8: Mismatched Libidos in Relationships

Sexual desire is a natural and vital aspect of most romantic relationships. However, it is rare for both partners to have perfectly aligned levels of sexual desire at all times. Differences in libido—one partner has a higher or lower desire for sex—are common, but they can create tension, frustration, and feelings of disconnection if not addressed openly. While mismatched libidos are normal, they can be emotionally and physically challenging to navigate. In this chapter, we will explore the reasons behind libido differences, how to foster understanding and communication around sexual desires, and practical strategies for reconnecting when libido differences arise.

When She Wants More, or Less: Navigating Mismatched Sexual Desire

The Reality of Mismatched Libidos

It's common for couples to experience differences in their levels of sexual desire. In some relationships, one partner may want sex more frequently, while the other may desire it less often. These mismatches are perfectly normal but can lead to feelings of rejection, frustration, or pressure if not handled openly and respectfully.

For the partner with the higher libido, it can feel like the other is no longer attracted to them or doesn't want to connect. Conversely, the partner with the lower libido might feel overwhelmed by expectations or guilt for not wanting sex as frequently. These differing needs can result in emotional distance or even resentment if not addressed constructively.

Common Scenarios Include:

<u>She Wants More</u>: Your partner might have a higher sex drive than you, leaving you feeling pressured or unsure of how to satisfy her needs while maintaining your comfort.

<u>She Wants Less</u>: If you have a higher libido than your partner, you might feel neglected or unwanted, causing frustration or insecurity.

The key to overcoming this mismatch is understanding that sexual desire fluctuates naturally and doesn't reflect how much love or attraction exists in the relationship.

Exercise 1: Reflecting on Your Libido

Assess Your Libido: Take a moment to reflect on your sexual desire. Do you find yourself wanting sex more or less than your partner? How does that make you feel, and how does it impact your relationship?

Recognize Your Partner's Perspective: Empathize with your partner's position. If they want sex more frequently than you, understand that this doesn't mean they are dissatisfied with the relationship—it's simply their natural desire. If they want less, recognize that it doesn't mean they're less attracted to you.

Accept the Mismatch: Write down one positive thing about your relationship outside of sex. This will help you see that mismatched libidos are just one aspect of a broader, healthy relationship.

Understanding Sexual Rhythms: Navigating Fluctuations in Desire

Mismatched libidos can manifest in many ways. Sometimes, one partner has a consistently higher sex drive, while the other has a lower or more fluctuating desire for sexual activity. At other times, the balance of desire may shift due to life events, stress, or hormonal changes. Regardless of the situation, it is essential to approach libido differences with empathy, patience, and a willingness to communicate openly.

1. Libido as a Spectrum, Not a Constant

Sexual desire is not static; it fluctuates over time and is influenced by a wide range of factors, including age, health, stress, relationship dynamics, and personal experiences. Rather than viewing libido as a fixed trait, it is more helpful to see it as a spectrum that changes throughout life. This perspective helps both partners to avoid making assumptions or judgments about their partner's desire levels.

External Influences on Libido: External factors such as work stress, financial concerns, health issues, or exhaustion can temporarily lower sexual desire. For example, someone dealing with a major life stressor might experience a significant drop in libido for a time, even if they are typically highly sexual.

Hormonal Fluctuations: Hormones also play a critical role in libido. For women, hormonal changes related to menstruation, pregnancy, postpartum recovery, and menopause can lead to variations in sexual desire. For men, testosterone levels and age-related hormonal changes can also impact libido over time.

2. Common Causes of Mismatched Libidos

Understanding the root causes of mismatched libidos is key to healthily addressing the issue. Some of the most common causes include:

Stress and Anxiety: Stressful life events or chronic stress can significantly impact a person's sex drive. Anxiety about work, finances, health, or the relationship itself can diminish desire or have sex feel like an added pressure.

Emotional Disconnect: Emotional intimacy plays a significant role in physical desire. If one partner feels emotionally distant or neglected, they may experience a decrease in sexual desire as a result. On the other hand, for some, sex may be a way to re-establish emotional closeness, creating a dynamic where one partner seeks more sex while the other pulls away.

Health and Medications: Physical health can also affect libido. Certain medications, such as antidepressants or blood pressure medications, may lower sex drive as a side effect. Additionally, health conditions like fatigue, chronic illness, or pain can decrease sexual interest.

Differing Sex Drives: Sometimes, partners have different natural baselines for sexual desire. One partner may have a higher sex drive, while the other naturally desires less frequent sexual activity. These differences are often hardwired and not necessarily caused by external factors.

3. The Emotional Impact of Mismatched Libidos

When partners experience mismatched libidos, it's not uncommon for both to feel a range of emotions. The partner with the higher libido may feel rejected, frustrated, or undesired, while the partner with the lower libido may feel guilty, pressured, or inadequate. These emotional responses can create a cycle of frustration and resentment if not addressed through open communication.

Feelings of Rejection: The partner with the higher libido may interpret their partner's lack of desire as a personal rejection, leading to feelings of insecurity or self-doubt. They may question if their partner still finds them attractive or is still invested in the relationship.

Pressure and Guilt: The partner with the lower libido may feel pressured to engage in sex to meet their partner's needs, even when they are not in the mood. This pressure can lead to feelings of guilt or resentment as they struggle to balance their own needs with their partner's expectations.

How to Navigate Libido Differences with Respect and Communication

The foundation of addressing mismatched libidos in any relationship is open, honest communication. Both partners need to feel safe discussing their desires, frustrations, and emotional responses without fear of judgment or blame. Here are some key strategies for improving communication and navigating sexual desire differences.

1. Start with Compassion and Empathy

Approach conversations about libido differences with empathy and a willingness to listen. Both partners are likely experiencing complex emotions—frustrations, guilt, or confusion—and it's essential to create a space where both parties feel heard and understood.

<u>Avoid Blame</u>: Rather than blaming your partner for the mismatch in libido, approach the conversation as a team. Use "I" statements rather than "you" statements to express your feelings. For example, instead of saying, "You never want to have sex," say, "I've noticed that our sex drives seem different, and I'd like to talk about how we can address this together."

<u>Acknowledge Emotions</u>: Acknowledge that both partners' feelings are valid. The partner with the higher libido may feel rejected, while the partner with the lower libido may feel pressured or overwhelmed. By validating each other's emotions, you can foster a sense of mutual understanding.

2. Explore Underlying Causes

Once you've established open communication, work together to explore the underlying causes of libido differences. Ask questions like:

Are there external stressors affecting one partner's sex drive?

Are there emotional issues within the relationship that need to be addressed?

Are physical health or medications playing a role in diminished desire?

Is there a disconnect in how each partner approaches emotional intimacy?

By identifying the potential root causes of mismatched libidos, you can begin to address those factors and find ways to reconnect.

Exercise 2: Understanding Your Partner's Sexual Rhythm

Track Fluctuations Together: Over the course of a month, keep a casual journal of your sexual desire levels. Afterward, compare it with your partner's to see how your libidos align or differ during different times of the month or in response to specific life events (e.g., work stress, vacations, health changes).

Respect Natural Differences: Acknowledge that libido fluctuations are natural and that it's okay for you and your partner to experience different sexual rhythms. Write down one thing you appreciate about your partner's unique sexual rhythm, like their spontaneity, tenderness, or playfulness.

Reconnecting Sexually: Finding Harmony When Libido Differences Exist

While communication is key, it's also important to implement practical strategies that can help partners reconnect sexually, even when their libidos don't align perfectly. Here are some approaches to help bridge the gap between different levels of sexual desire.

1. Redefine Intimacy Beyond Penetrative Sex

One of the most effective ways to navigate mismatched libidos is to expand your definition of intimacy beyond penetrative sex. For many couples, physical intimacy becomes equated with sex, but there are many other ways to connect and maintain closeness, including cuddling, kissing, holding hands, and non-sexual touch.

<u>Non-Sexual Intimacy</u>: Engage in activities that build physical closeness without the expectation of sex. Non-sexual touch can help maintain intimacy and reduce feelings of pressure or rejection. This can include massage, cuddling while watching a movie, or taking a bath together.

<u>Mutual Pleasure</u>: Explore other forms of mutual pleasure that don't require penetrative sex, such as oral sex, mutual masturbation, or simply enjoying each other's bodies in a way that feels good for both partners.

2. Schedule Intimacy

While scheduling sex may seem unromantic, it can actually be a helpful strategy for couples with mismatched libidos. By agreeing on specific times for intimacy, both partners can anticipate and prepare for the experience. This can help reduce the pressure to spontaneously initiate sex, which can be a source of anxiety for both partners.

Set Expectations: Scheduling intimacy allows both partners to set realistic expectations about when and how often they'll engage in sexual activity. This helps create a sense of mutual understanding and reduces the risk of one partner feeling pressured to have sex when they're not in the mood.

Create a Ritual: Use scheduled intimacy as an opportunity to create a ritual or routine that both partners enjoy. This could involve a date night, a relaxing evening together, or any other activity that helps set the mood and build emotional connection before engaging in physical intimacy.

3. Focus on Foreplay and Emotional Connection

For many couples, mismatched libidos are rooted in a lack of emotional intimacy or insufficient focus on foreplay. One partner may need more emotional connection or physical stimulation to become aroused, while the other may become aroused more quickly. Focusing on emotional connection and extended foreplay can help both partners feel more engaged in the sexual experience.

Extended Foreplay: Spend more time on foreplay to build anticipation and arousal for both partners. This can include kissing, touching, talking, or engaging in activities that foster emotional and physical connection.

Emotional Connection: Work on building emotional intimacy outside of the bedroom. Engage in deep conversations, spend quality time together, and strengthen your bond as a couple. When emotional intimacy is strong, physical intimacy often follows more naturally.

4. Seek Professional Help if Needed

If mismatched libidos continue to create tension in the relationship, it may be helpful to seek the guidance of a sex therapist or couples' counselor. A professional can help both partners explore the underlying issues contributing to libido differences and offer tailored strategies for improving communication, intimacy, and sexual satisfaction.

Sex Therapy: A sex therapist can help couples navigate the emotional and psychological aspects of mismatched libidos, offering tools to improve communication and reconnect physically.

Couples Counseling: If there are deeper emotional or relational issues affecting sexual desire, couples counseling can help address those issues in a supportive environment.

Exercise 3: Reconnecting Through Intimacy

Plan an Intimacy Date Night: Set aside a night for non-sexual intimacy. Plan activities like giving each other massages, taking a bath together or just spending time cuddling. This helps reconnect physically without pressure.

Create an Excitement Jar: Each partner can write down a few intimate activities or fantasies they want to explore. It can be something new or an old favorite. Place these ideas in a jar, and randomly choose one to try together on date nights. This introduces novelty and anticipation, which can help bridge libido differences.

Finding Balance and Connection with Mismatched Libidos

Mismatched libidos are a normal and natural part of many relationships. Rather than viewing these differences as a source of conflict, couples can approach them as an opportunity to deepen their understanding of each other's needs, desires, and emotional landscapes. Through open communication, empathy, and practical strategies for maintaining intimacy, partners can find ways to bridge the gap and enjoy a fulfilling, connected sexual relationship— even when their libidos don't always align.

By focusing on emotional intimacy, exploring new ways of experiencing physical pleasure, and addressing underlying issues, couples can navigate libido differences with compassion and understanding, ultimately strengthening their bond.

PART IV: Sexual Experiences and Fantasies

Sexual fantasies are a natural and healthy aspect of human sexuality, allowing individuals to explore their desires, preferences, and curiosities in a safe, imaginative way. However, many men feel a deep sense of shame surrounding their fantasies, especially if they believe their desires deviate from societal norms or are considered taboo. This shame can create a disconnect between their sexual desires and their relationships, often preventing them from fully embracing their fantasies or sharing them with their partners.

In this chapter, we will explore the roots of shame surrounding sexual fantasies, why it is important to normalize and accept these desires, and how to communicate fantasies with a partner in a way that fosters trust, openness, and mutual respect.

Chapter 9: Sexual Fantasies, Infidelity Fantasies, and Shame

Sexual fantasies are a natural and healthy aspect of human sexuality, allowing individuals to explore their desires, preferences, and curiosities in a safe, imaginative way. However, many men feel a deep sense of shame surrounding their fantasies, especially if they believe their desires deviate from societal norms or are considered taboo. This shame can create a disconnect between their sexual desires and their relationships, often preventing them from fully embracing their fantasies or sharing them with their partners.

In this chapter, we will explore the roots of shame surrounding sexual fantasies, why it is important to normalize and accept these desires, and how to communicate fantasies with a partner in a way that fosters trust, openness, and mutual respect.

Understanding Sexual Fantasies and Why They Matter

Sexual fantasies are mental explorations of erotic or sexual scenarios that may or may not align with a person's real-life experiences. These fantasies allow individuals to express parts of their sexuality that they might not feel comfortable acting on in reality or that they find pleasurable to imagine. For many people, sexual fantasies are an essential part of maintaining a healthy sexual relationship and can enhance sexual satisfaction

1. Why Sexual Fantasies Are Important

Sexual fantasies serve several key functions, both for individuals and within relationships. Some of the most significant reasons why fantasies are important include:

<u>Exploration of Desires</u>: Fantasies allow people to safely explore desires, kinks, or preferences without necessarily needing to act them out in real life. This can be empowering, as it enables individuals to express their sexual desires without feeling constrained by societal norms or personal inhibitions.

<u>Enhancing Sexual Arousal</u>: For many men, sexual fantasies can enhance arousal, either during solo sexual activities like masturbation or in partnered experiences. Fantasizing about specific scenarios or desires can make sex more exciting and increase overall satisfaction.

<u>Emotional Release</u>: Fantasies provide a safe space for emotional release, especially when it comes to desires or impulses that might be considered taboo. By imagining these scenarios, men can express aspects of themselves that they may feel are repressed or unacceptable in other areas of life.

Why Men Feel Ashamed of Their Fantasies

How Shame Develops Around Sexual Fantasies

Men often internalize shame about their sexual fantasies due to societal and cultural pressures. From an early age, men are taught that certain desires or fantasies are "acceptable," while others are seen as deviant or abnormal. Pornography, societal standards, and rigid gender roles can reinforce the idea that anything outside of "vanilla" sex is wrong or perverse.

This internalization of sexual norms leads to feelings of guilt, embarrassment, or even self-disgust when a man's fantasies don't align with what he perceives to be "normal." Many men suppress or hide these desires, fearing that they are alone in their thoughts or that expressing them would lead to rejection or ridicule.

1. Societal Norms and Expectations

One of the primary sources of shame around sexual fantasies is societal norms. Mainstream media, cultural expectations, and even pornography often present a limited and sanitized version of sexuality, leaving little room for sexual expression that deviates from the "norm." Men are often bombarded with messages about what is considered "acceptable" or "normal" sexual behavior, leading them to internalize these narrow views.

<u>Fear of Judgment</u>: Many men fear that their fantasies will be judged as deviant, immoral, or perverse, particularly if those fantasies involve non-traditional scenarios like power dynamics, role play, or group sex. This fear of judgment can cause men to feel isolated and ashamed of their desires, believing that they are alone in their fantasies.

<u>Cultural Taboos</u>: Certain fantasies are considered more taboo than others based on cultural or religious values. For

example, fantasies involving BDSM, submission, or non-monogamous scenarios are often viewed as inappropriate or unhealthy by mainstream society. This cultural taboo can make it difficult for men to accept their fantasies, even if they are normal and consensual.

2. Personal Insecurities and Self-Worth

Men who struggle with self-esteem or self-worth may feel particularly vulnerable when it comes to their sexual fantasies. They may worry that their desires make them less "manly" or that their fantasies indicate some kind of flaw or deficiency in their character. This fear of inadequacy can lead to deep feelings of shame, making it difficult to embrace their sexual fantasies openly.

<u>Internal Conflict</u>: Men may experience internal conflict between their fantasies and their self-image, especially if their desires contradict the way they want to see themselves. For instance, a man who views himself as dominant or assertive may feel shame if he fantasizes about submission or being vulnerable during sex.

<u>Body Image and Performance Anxiety</u>: Men who experience body image issues or performance anxiety may also feel ashamed of their fantasies if they believe they don't "deserve" to explore their desires. They may worry that their physical appearance or sexual abilities aren't good enough to live up to the fantasies they envision.

3. The Impact of Pornography

While pornography can serve as an outlet for sexual exploration, it can also contribute to feelings of shame or guilt, especially when it comes to sexual fantasies. Men who consume pornography may compare their fantasies to the exaggerated or unrealistic portrayals of sex they see on screen, leading to insecurity or confusion about their own desires.

<u>Comparing Fantasies to Porn</u>: Pornography often presents idealized, unrealistic depictions of sexual encounters, which can distort men's perceptions of their own fantasies. They may feel that their desires are "too weird" or "not exciting enough" compared to the fantasies depicted in porn, leading to feelings of inadequacy.

<u>Reinforcing Shame</u>: Some men may use pornography as a way to indulge in fantasies they feel ashamed of, only to experience guilt or shame after viewing it. This cycle of indulging in and then repressing fantasies can create a negative relationship with sexual desire, reinforcing feelings of shame and self-judgment.

Exercise 1: Confronting Shame

Identify Your Shame: Write down the fantasies that make you feel ashamed. Be specific about why you feel these desires are "wrong" or "deviant."

Challenge Negative Beliefs: Next to each fantasy, write down a counter-narrative. For example, if you feel ashamed of a dominance fantasy, challenge it by writing, "It's okay to enjoy role-playing in a consensual, respectful relationship. Fantasies are a normal part of sexual expression."

<u>*Reflect on Cultural Influences*</u>: Consider where your feelings of shame come from—are they rooted in societal standards, religious beliefs, or past experiences? Acknowledging the external influences on your shame can help you recognize that these feelings aren't an inherent reflection of your worth or character.

The Emotional Impact of Shame

When men feel ashamed of their fantasies, it can lead to emotional distress, anxiety, and a sense of isolation. Over time, this shame can erode self-esteem and cause men to distance themselves from their own sexuality, making it difficult to enjoy or explore their desires fully.

Key Consequences Include:

<u>Emotional Repression</u>: Men may repress their sexual desires, causing feelings of frustration or dissatisfaction in their relationships.

<u>Fear of Rejection</u>: The fear of being judged or rejected by a partner can prevent men from being open about their fantasies, leading to a lack of emotional and sexual intimacy.

<u>Disconnect from Self</u>: Men may feel disconnected from their authentic sexual selves, suppressing desires that could otherwise enhance their sexual and emotional well-being.

Why Men Fantasize About Infidelity

The Psychology Behind Cheating Fantasies

Infidelity fantasies often stem from complex psychological and emotional desires. These fantasies don't necessarily indicate a desire to cheat in real life, but they can reveal deeper needs or unaddressed issues within a relationship.

Key Reasons for Infidelity Fantasies:

<u>The Thrill of the Forbidden</u>: For some men, fantasizing about cheating provides a sense of excitement or thrill that can be missing in a long-term relationship. The idea of engaging in something "forbidden" can heighten arousal, even if they have no intention of acting on it.

<u>Boredom or Routine</u>: Over time, relationships can fall into a routine, and the sexual excitement that once existed may fade. Infidelity fantasies can arise as a way to mentally escape this monotony, seeking the excitement and novelty that new relationships often bring.

<u>Unmet Emotional or Sexual Needs</u>: Sometimes, these fantasies point to unmet needs—emotional, physical, or both. If a man feels disconnected from his partner or unsatisfied in the relationship, his mind might wander to scenarios where he imagines receiving what he's missing elsewhere.

It's important to note that fantasizing about infidelity doesn't mean a man is inherently unhappy in his relationship. In many cases, these thoughts are simply a reflection of human nature—the desire for novelty, excitement, or even emotional validation.

The Role of Power and Control

For some men, fantasies of infidelity are tied to feelings of power or control. Being desired by someone outside the relationship can boost self-esteem or serve as a validation of one's attractiveness. This can be particularly appealing during times of insecurity or doubt about one's desirability.

Exercise 2: Understanding Your Infidelity Fantasies

Write Down the Fantasy: Without judgment, write down the specifics of your infidelity fantasy. What is it about the scenario that excites you? Is it the novelty, the secrecy, the power dynamic, or something else?

Reflect on What the Fantasy Reveals: Consider what your fantasy might be telling you about your current relationship or emotional state. Are you feeling bored, disconnected, or seeking validation? Understanding the underlying reasons behind the fantasy can help you address those needs within your relationship.

Normalizing Sexual Fantasies: A Healthy Part of Desire

Why Having Fantasies Is Normal and Healthy

Sexual fantasies are a natural part of human sexuality. They allow people to explore desires, push boundaries, and experience excitement without necessarily acting on those fantasies in real life. Fantasies can provide a safe mental space to explore new dynamics, roles, or scenarios, adding richness to one's sexual imagination.

Rather than viewing fantasies as something to be ashamed of, it's important to understand that they are a normal and healthy part of sexual desire. Everyone has fantasies, and they don't have to reflect real-life desires or behaviors. For example, someone might fantasize about a scenario they would never want to happen in real life, and that's perfectly normal.

1. Understanding that Fantasies Are Not Reality

One key point to remember about sexual fantasies is that they don't always mirror real-life desires. A man may fantasize about a particular scenario without actually intending to act on it. Fantasies are often symbolic or metaphorical, representing various emotions, such as the desire for control or the need for openness and emotional expression.

<u>Fantasy vs. Reality</u>: It's important to distinguish between fantasy and reality. Many fantasies are rooted in exploring ideas that may not align with one's real-life values or actions. For example, a man may fantasize about a consensual power exchange scenario without wanting to live out those dynamics in his everyday life.

Giving Yourself Permission to Fantasize: Recognizing that
fantasies are not binding or definitive allows men to permit
themselves to explore their desires without guilt.
Embracing the fact that fantasies are a healthy outlet for
imagination and curiosity can reduce feelings of shame.

2. Embracing Your Desires Without Judgment

Releasing shame around sexual fantasies requires self-
compassion and acceptance. Men should aim to embrace
their fantasies without self-judgment, acknowledging that
their desires are unique to them and do not make them
inherently flawed or wrong.

Self-Compassion: Practice self-compassion by reminding
yourself that everyone has sexual fantasies, and there is no
universal standard for what is "normal." Instead of
criticizing yourself for your desires, try to view them with
curiosity and acceptance.

Exploring Desires Safely: If there are fantasies that you're
curious about exploring in real life, do so in a way that
aligns with your boundaries and values. Ensure that any
real-life exploration is consensual, safe, and rooted in
mutual respect.

3. Recognizing Common Fantasies

Many men feel isolated in their fantasies, believing that
their desires are unique or deviant. However, studies show
that many sexual fantasies are incredibly common and
shared by a wide range of individuals. Some of the most
common fantasies include:

Power Dynamics: Fantasies involving dominance and submission are among the most common, with many people fantasizing about giving up control or taking charge in a sexual scenario.

Group Sex: Fantasies about group sex, threesomes, or multiple partners are also common, even if they don't align with real-life preferences or relationship dynamics.

Role Play: Fantasies about role play or taking on different personas in the bedroom allow individuals to explore aspects of their sexuality that may be repressed in their everyday lives.

By recognizing that others share many sexual fantasies, men can begin to feel less isolated and ashamed of their desires.

Benefits of Embracing Sexual Fantasies:

Sexual fantasies are a natural part of human sexuality and can be a powerful tool for enhancing intimacy, creativity, and self-awareness. Far from being something to be ashamed of, fantasies offer insight into our desires, help us explore boundaries, and deepen our connection with ourselves and our partners. Embracing sexual fantasies in a healthy way and openly can lead to numerous benefits for both individuals and relationships.

Enhances Sexual Enjoyment: Fantasies can enhance sexual arousal, making experiences more exciting and pleasurable.

<u>Expands Intimacy</u>: Sharing fantasies with a partner can deepen emotional and sexual intimacy, creating a stronger bond through trust and openness.

<u>Improves Self-Awareness</u>: Exploring fantasies helps you better understand your desires, allowing you to embrace your sexual individuality more fully.

Exploring Fantasies Safely

While fantasies are healthy, it's important to explore them in a way that respects your boundaries and those of your partner. Not every fantasy needs to be acted upon—sometimes, just acknowledging the fantasy is enough. However, if you and your partner are open to exploring certain fantasies, ensure that you approach them with clear communication, mutual consent, and respect.

Safe Exploration Tips:

<u>Start with Conversation</u>: Before acting on a fantasy, talk about it with your partner. Make sure both of you feel comfortable and excited about the idea.

<u>Set Boundaries</u>: Discuss any limits or boundaries before engaging in any new activities. Consent is key to safe exploration.

<u>Understand That Fantasies Are Just That</u>: Some fantasies are best left as fantasies. Not everything that turns you on mentally needs to be acted out physically.

Exercise 3: Embracing Fantasies Without Shame

List Your Fantasies: Write down any sexual fantasies you have, without judgment. Allow yourself to acknowledge these desires as a normal part of your sexuality.

Rank Comfort Levels: Next to each fantasy, rate how comfortable you are with the idea of exploring it. This helps you identify which fantasies you might want to discuss with a partner and which ones you prefer to keep private.

Practice Affirmation: Write a positive affirmation about your sexual desires. For example, "It's okay for me to have fantasies, and they are a healthy part of my sexuality."

Sharing Fantasies with a Partner: Opening Up Without Fear

How to Bring Up Fantasies in a Relationship

While it's normal to feel hesitant about sharing sexual fantasies with a partner, open communication is key to building a trusting and fulfilling sexual relationship. When fantasies are shared in a supportive, non-judgmental environment, they can foster intimacy, spark new forms of connection, and create opportunities for deeper exploration.

1. How to Share Your Fantasies

Sharing sexual fantasies with a partner requires a foundation of trust and openness. It's crucial to approach these conversations with sensitivity, ensuring that both partners feel safe, respected, and understood throughout the discussion.

<u>Choose the Right Time</u>: Timing is important when discussing sexual fantasies. Make sure to have this conversation when both you and your partner are relaxed and open to discussion rather than during a stressful moment or right before sex.

<u>Use "I" Statements</u>: When sharing fantasies, focus on your own experiences and desires by using "I" statements. For example, instead of saying, "You never want to try this," say, "I've been thinking about this fantasy, and I'd like to explore it with you."

<u>Be Open to Their Response</u>: Your partner's reaction may vary depending on their comfort level with the fantasy. Be open to their response and allow them to express their feelings without pressuring them into accepting or participating in the fantasy.

2. How to Respond When a Partner Shares Fantasies

If your partner shares their sexual fantasies with you, it's important to approach the conversation with openness and understanding. Respond with empathy and curiosity even if the fantasy is something you're not comfortable with or have never considered.

<u>Validate Their Vulnerability</u>: Let your partner explain their fantasy without interrupting or reacting negatively. Acknowledge the courage it took for your partner to share their fantasy with you. Let them know that you appreciate their openness and are interested in understanding their desires, even if they differ from yours.

<u>Ask Questions</u>: If you're unsure about the fantasy, ask questions to better understand what excites them about it.

<u>Explore Together</u>: If the fantasy resonates with you, consider discussing how you can explore it together in a way that feels comfortable for both of you. This may involve setting boundaries, experimenting with role play, or simply discussing the fantasy to better understand its meaning.

<u>Respect Boundaries</u>: If the fantasy doesn't align with your comfort level, it's okay to set boundaries. However, try to do so in a way that is respectful and affirming of your partner's desires. Instead of dismissing the fantasy outright, discuss alternatives or ways to meet each other's needs in a way that feels mutually satisfying.

Exercise 4: Sharing Fantasies with Your Partner

<u>Start Small</u>: If you're nervous about sharing your fantasies, start by discussing a fantasy that's less intense or personal. Gauge your partner's reaction and build from there.

<u>Use Media as a Gateway</u>: Sometimes, watching a movie or reading erotica together can be a way to introduce the idea of fantasies. This can lead to a natural conversation about desires without feeling like you're putting yourself on the spot.

<u>Check-In with Your Partner</u>: After sharing your fantasy, check in with your partner to see how they're feeling. Ask if they have any fantasies they'd like to share or explore together.

Managing Infidelity Fantasies: Acknowledging Desires Without Acting on Them

Why Acting on Infidelity Fantasies Is Harmful

While fantasizing about infidelity is a common and sometimes harmless mental exercise, acting on those fantasies can have severe consequences. Cheating can break trust, cause emotional damage, and lead to the breakdown of a relationship. It's essential to acknowledge these desires and address what they reveal about your relationship without crossing the line into infidelity.

How to Acknowledge These Fantasies Without Acting on Them

Instead of feeling guilty or suppressing your fantasies, learn to acknowledge them in a healthy way. Fantasies are a natural part of sexual expression and don't have to dictate your actions.

Steps to Acknowledge Infidelity Fantasies:

<u>Recognize Them as Normal</u>: It's important to remember that having fantasies is normal and doesn't automatically mean you want to act on them. These thoughts can be a way to explore different aspects of your sexuality or unmet needs without jeopardizing your relationship.

Avoid Guilt or Shame: Don't shame yourself for having these thoughts. Fantasizing is not the same as cheating, and feeling guilty will only add unnecessary emotional stress.

Use Fantasies as Insight: Consider what your fantasies might be telling you about your relationship. Are there areas where you feel emotionally or sexually unfulfilled? Use this insight to initiate positive changes in your relationship.

Exercise 5: Managing Infidelity Fantasies

Acknowledge Without Judgment: The next time you have an infidelity fantasy, take a moment to acknowledge it without guilt. Allow yourself to explore the fantasy in your mind without feeling pressure to act on it.

Identify Unmet Needs: Reflect on this fantasy and if it points to any unmet emotional or physical needs in your relationship. Write down areas where you feel unfulfilled and consider ways to address these issues with your partner.

Reigniting Desire Within Your Relationship

Turning Infidelity Fantasies into a Positive Force

One of the key challenges in relationships is maintaining sexual desire over time. As routines set in and life's responsibilities take center stage, sexual passion can sometimes take a backseat. However, by addressing the underlying desires that fuel fantasies of infidelity, you can reignite desire in your relationship and strengthen your emotional and sexual bond. Rather than viewing infidelity fantasies as a sign of dissatisfaction, use them as an opportunity to reignite the passion within your current relationship. These fantasies often concern novelty, excitement, and emotional connection—which can be cultivated within your relationship.

Ways to Channel Fantasies into Your Relationship:

1. Breaking Out of Routine

Long-term relationships can fall into a comfortable but predictable rhythm. Breaking out of this routine and introducing new elements of surprise and excitement is essential to reignite desire.

<u>Try New Activities Together</u>: A new hobby, vacation, or date night, trying new activities together can create a sense of adventure and connection that rekindles the spark in your relationship.

<u>Revisit What You Loved Early in the Relationship</u>: Sometimes, looking back at the early days of your relationship can reignite passion. Think about the things you used to do together when you first fell in love, and make an effort to recreate those moments.

2. Exploring New Sexual Experiences

Sexual exploration doesn't have to end just because a relationship has entered the long-term phase. Trying new sexual experiences together can inject excitement and curiosity into your relationship, helping both partners feel more connected and desired.

<u>Spice Up Your Sex Life</u>: If boredom or routine is contributing to your fantasies, take steps to bring excitement back into your sexual relationship. This could involve trying new positions, exploring role-play, or experimenting with fantasies that you and your partner are both comfortable with.

<u>Communicate Sexual Desires</u>: Talk openly with your partner about any new sexual desires or fantasies you'd like to explore together.

<u>Focus on Pleasure Over Performance</u>: Let go of any pressure to "perform" in the bedroom and instead focus on mutual pleasure. When both partners feel relaxed and open, sex becomes more enjoyable and intimate.

3. Prioritizing Emotional Connection

Physical intimacy is closely tied to emotional intimacy, especially in long-term relationships. Strengthening your emotional connection can deepen your sexual experiences and reignite desire.

<u>Practice Openness</u>: Be open with your partner about your emotions, fears, and needs. Practicing openness builds trust and creates a deeper emotional bond that translates into greater intimacy in the bedroom.

Show Appreciation: Sometimes infidelity fantasies arise from a lack of emotional intimacy. Expressing gratitude and appreciation for your partner can help foster emotional closeness. Small acts of kindness, compliments, and gestures of love go a long way in keeping the connection strong.

Communicate Openly with Your Partner: If your fantasies point to unmet needs, have an open and honest conversation with your partner. Talk about what you both desire and how you can make your sex life more fulfilling. You don't have to reveal your infidelity fantasies directly, but addressing the underlying issues can help.

Embracing and Sharing Fantasies Without Shame

Sexual fantasies are a natural and healthy part of human sexuality. By embracing these desires without shame, men can begin to explore their sexual character more fully and build deeper connections with their partners. Normalizing fantasies, by either aligning them with societal norms or not, allows men to reclaim their sexuality and feel empowered by their desires rather than burdened by them.

Infidelity fantasies are also a natural part of human sexuality, often driven by boredom, unmet needs, or the desire for novelty. While these fantasies can feel troubling, they don't have to be a source of guilt or a precursor to cheating. By acknowledging your desires, exploring what they reveal about your relationship, and channeling that energy back into your partnership, you can reignite passion and build a stronger, more fulfilling connection.

Remember, fantasies are not inherently harmful—they can offer valuable insights into what you desire and what your relationship might need. Use them as a tool to understand yourself and your partner more deeply rather than a reason to act outside the boundaries of trust. Open communication with a partner about fantasies can lead to greater trust, intimacy, and shared exploration, ultimately enriching the sexual and emotional connection between partners.

Chapter 10: Kinks, Fetishes, and Exploration

Kinks and fetishes are a natural part of human sexuality, often allowing individuals to explore unique aspects of desire and pleasure. For many men, these preferences are deeply ingrained in their sexual expression, offering a source of arousal, excitement, and fulfillment. Yet, due to societal taboos and personal insecurities, many men feel hesitant or even ashamed to discuss their kinks or fetishes openly. This silence can create distance in relationships and prevent individuals from fully embracing their sexuality.

What Are Kinks and Fetishes?

Before diving into why men hesitate to discuss these desires, it's important to clarify what we mean by kinks and fetishes.

Kinks refer to any unconventional sexual preferences or practices that fall outside of traditional sexual norms but are consensual and safe. These could include things like BDSM (bondage, discipline, dominance, submission, sadism, and masochism), role play, voyeurism, or other non-traditional acts that bring sexual pleasure.

Fetishes are specific, often intense sexual attractions to objects, body parts, or scenarios that may not traditionally be considered sexual. Fetishes might focus on feet, leather, or specific clothing items. For someone with a fetish, these objects or scenarios are often essential to sexual arousal or satisfaction.

Both kinks and fetishes can add variety, excitement, and depth to sexual experiences. However, because they often deviate from mainstream expectations, discussing these desires openly can feel intimidating.

Unspoken Desires: Why Men Often Hide Their Kinks and Fetishes

The Pressure to Conform

Kinks and fetishes, while a natural part of human sexuality, often remain hidden due to societal pressures and misconceptions. Men are frequently taught that sexual desires should fit within a narrow range of "acceptable" activities, leading to shame or embarrassment when their preferences fall outside these perceived norms.

This reluctance to talk about kinks and fetishes often stems from fear of judgment or rejection by a partner or society at large. Many men worry that revealing their desires will be met with disgust or that it will damage their relationship. As a result, these desires are often kept secret, leading to frustration, emotional distance, or feelings of isolation within a relationship.

1. Societal Judgment and Taboos

Kinks and fetishes often carry a stigma, as society tends to equate sexual "normalcy" with conventional, vanilla sexual practices. Anything that deviates from this norm is often viewed as strange, perverse, or even shameful. Men who internalize these societal judgments may fear that their desires will be met with ridicule or disgust if they share them.

<u>Fear of Being Labeled as Deviant</u>: Many men worry that expressing their kinks or fetishes will lead to them being labeled as deviant or abnormal, especially if their desires are considered taboo. This fear of judgment can cause men to keep their preferences hidden, leading to internalized shame.

<u>Cultural and Religious Expectations</u>: In some cultures or religious contexts, kinks and fetishes are seen as sinful or immoral. These values can create additional pressure for men to suppress or deny their sexual preferences, reinforcing the idea that their desires are wrong.

2. Fear of Rejection

One of the most common fears men face when discussing kinks or fetishes with a partner is the fear of rejection. They may worry that sharing their desires will cause their partner to feel uncomfortable, lose attraction, or even end the relationship. This fear can be especially intense if the kink or fetish is integral to their sexual identity.

<u>Risk of Relationship Conflict</u>: Men may hesitate to share their desires out of fear that it will cause tension in the relationship, especially if their partner is not open to exploring the same kinks or fetishes. This can lead to feelings of isolation or frustration, as men are left suppressing a core part of their sexual expression.

Insecurity About Desirability: For some men, there is an underlying fear that sharing their kinks or fetishes will make them less desirable to their partner. They may worry that their partner will see them differently or lose respect for them after learning about their desires.

3. Lack of Understanding of Desires

Another reason men may hesitate to discuss their kinks or fetishes is that they may not fully understand them. It can be difficult to explain desires that feel complex, confusing, or even contradictory to one's self-image. Men may feel unsure of how to articulate their kinks or fetishes in a way that their partner can understand.

Internal Conflict: Some men experience an internal conflict between their sexual preferences and how they view themselves. For example, a man who values control and assertiveness in his daily life might struggle to accept a submissive kink. This conflict can make it hard to open up about these desires without feeling a sense of discomfort or shame.

Difficulty Defining Desires: Because kinks and fetishes can be highly specific and personal, men may not always have the language or framework to clearly define what they want. This lack of clarity can make it challenging to start a conversation with a partner about exploring these desires.

How Silence Can Harm Relationships

When men keep their kinks or fetishes hidden, it can lead to emotional strain. Not only does the individual feel disconnected from their partner, but the relationship can suffer from a lack of openness. This secrecy can create tension and prevent both partners from fully enjoying their sexual connection.

Consequences of Unspoken Desires Include:

<u>Resentment</u>: Over time, hiding a significant part of your sexuality can lead to resentment, either toward your partner or yourself, for not being able to explore what excites you.

<u>Emotional Distance</u>: Keeping desires hidden can create a barrier to emotional and sexual intimacy, making it harder to connect on a deeper level.

<u>Unfulfilled Needs</u>: When kinks or fetishes are kept in the shadows, men often feel unsatisfied in their sex lives, leading to frustration or a lack of fulfillment.

Exercise 1: Reflecting on Your Unspoken Desires

Identify Your Kinks or Fetishes: Write down any kinks or fetishes you have but haven't shared with a partner. Be honest with yourself about what turns you on without judging or censoring your desires.

Consider Why You Haven't Shared: Next to each desire, reflect on why you haven't shared it with your partner. Are you afraid of being judged? Do you worry it might damage the relationship? This can help you understand the barriers that are preventing open communication.

Reframe the Conversation: For each unspoken desire, write down a positive way to introduce it in conversation. For example, instead of saying, "I know this might sound weird, but…" you might say, "There's something I've been thinking about that could be really fun for us to try together."

Exploring Kinks Safely: Introducing Desires with Clear Communication

How to Introduce Kinks or Fetishes to a Partner

Introducing a kink or fetish into a relationship can be intimidating, but it's important to approach the conversation with honesty, clear communication, and respect for boundaries. Many partners are open to exploring new things as long as the conversation feels safe and non-threatening. The key is creating a space where you and your partner feel comfortable expressing desires and limits.

Steps for Introducing a Kink or Fetish:

Choose the Right Time: Timing is everything when discussing sensitive topics. Make sure you bring up the conversation when both of you are relaxed and open to talking about sex rather than during a stressful or rushed moment.

Be Honest and Vulnerable: Explain that sharing this desire is important to you, and express your hope for a non-judgmental conversation. For example, "I've been thinking about something that excites me sexually, and I'd love to share it with you because I want us to feel close and connected."

Invite a Collaborative Approach: Frame the discussion to enhance your relationship rather than focus solely on your needs. Ask your partner how they feel about exploring the kink together and encourage them to share their desires.

Start Slow: If your partner is unsure or hesitant, suggest starting small. For example, if you're introducing a bondage kink, you might suggest using a silk scarf or light restraints instead of jumping into more advanced forms of play.

Setting Boundaries for Safe Exploration

Exploring kinks and fetishes can be a fun and rewarding experience, but it's important to set clear boundaries to ensure both partners feel comfortable and safe. Consent is crucial in any sexual exploration, especially when trying something new.

Key Steps for Safe Exploration:

Discuss Limits: Before trying anything new, discuss each other's boundaries. What are you both willing to explore? Are there off-limits activities? Clear communication ensures that both partners feel respected and secure.

Use Safe Words: For more intense kinks, especially those that involve power dynamics or physical restraint, agree on a safe word that either partner can use if they feel uncomfortable or want to stop. This creates a safety net for exploration.

<u>Check In Regularly</u>: During and after exploring a new kink or fetish, check in with your partner to see how they're feeling. Asking, "How are you enjoying this?" or "Is there anything you'd like to change?" helps maintain open communication and ensures mutual satisfaction.

Exercise 2: Preparing for the Conversation

<u>Write Down How You Want to Approach the Topic</u>: Practice how you might introduce your kink or fetish to your partner by writing down a few key points you want to address. For example, start by expressing your desire for a fun, respectful, and mutual exploration.

<u>List Boundaries</u>: Before the conversation, write down any boundaries or limits you have regarding the kink or fetish. This helps clarify what you're comfortable with and allows you to approach the conversation with clear expectations.

Getting Comfortable with Your Desires: Embracing Your Kinks Without Shame

Why Kinks and Fetishes Are Normal

Kinks and fetishes are more common than people often realize. A kink is simply any non-conventional sexual preference, while a fetish is a specific object or scenario that arouses someone sexually. These desires don't make you strange or deviant—they are just part of the broad spectrum of human sexuality. Many people have kinks or fetishes, whether they realize it or not.

Embracing your kinks or fetishes means understanding that they are a healthy part of your sexual expression. Rather than feeling ashamed, acknowledge that these desires are unique to you and can enhance your sex life when explored in a consensual and respectful way.

Overcoming Shame: Embracing Your Desires

To overcome the shame that often accompanies kinks and fetishes, it's essential to reframe the way you view your sexual desires. Kinks and fetishes are not signs of deviance or abnormality; they are a natural part of sexual diversity. By accepting your desires and recognizing that they are valid and healthy, you can begin to shed the layers of shame and embrace your sexuality with confidence.

1. Normalize Your Desires

One of the first steps to overcoming shame is to normalize your kinks or fetishes. Acknowledge that sexual diversity is part of what makes human sexuality rich and varied. Just because your desires don't align with mainstream sexual practices doesn't mean they are wrong or something to be hidden.

Acknowledge Sexual Diversity: People's sexual preferences exist on a wide spectrum, and kinks and fetishes are more common than you might think. Many individuals have specific desires or fantasies that fall outside the "norm." Acknowledging this diversity helps dismantle the idea that there is only one "correct" way to experience sexual pleasure.

<u>Recognize that Fantasies Are Not Realities</u>: Having a kink or fetish doesn't mean you need to act on every fantasy in real life. Many people enjoy the mental exploration of a kink or fetish without feeling the need to experience it physically. Recognizing this distinction can help reduce anxiety about your desires.

2. Let Go of Judgment and Guilt

Releasing judgment toward yourself is critical in overcoming shame. Your kinks or fetishes do not define your worth or character. Instead of viewing your desires as something to be ashamed of, reframe them as an integral part of your sexual individuality.

<u>Practice Self-Compassion</u>: Be kind to yourself when reflecting on your desires. Everyone has unique sexual preferences, and those preferences are not a reflection of your morality or self-worth. Instead of criticizing yourself for your desires, try to view them with curiosity and acceptance.

<u>Challenge Negative Beliefs</u>: If you hold negative beliefs about your kinks or fetishes, ask yourself where those beliefs come from. Were they shaped by societal messages, cultural expectations, or past experiences? Challenging these beliefs helps you create a new, more positive narrative about your sexuality.

3. Explore Your Desires Safely

If you want to explore your kinks or fetishes in real life, it's important to do so safely and consensually. Engaging in consensual play with a partner allows you to experience your desires in a way that aligns with your boundaries and comfort level.

<u>Set Clear Boundaries</u>: Before engaging in any kink or fetish play, establish clear boundaries with your partner. Make sure both of you understand what you are comfortable with and what is off-limits. This helps create a safe environment for exploration.

<u>Communicate Openly</u>: Keep the lines of communication open throughout your exploration. Check-in with your partner regularly to ensure that both of you are feeling comfortable and respected. Consent and mutual agreement are essential in any sexual activity, especially when exploring kinks or fetishes.

<u>Accept Your Sexuality</u>: The first step to embracing your kinks is accepting that they are a part of who you are. It's important to recognize that kinks and fetishes are not inherently bad—they are simply preferences that can be explored in safe, consensual environments.

<u>Challenge Negative Thoughts</u>: If you feel ashamed of your desires, challenge those feelings. Ask yourself why you feel that way and if those beliefs are based on societal norms rather than your own values.

<u>Find Community</u>: Many people feel more comfortable with their kinks or fetishes when they realize they aren't alone. Finding a supportive community online or in-person, can

help normalize your desires and provide a sense of belonging.

Exercise 3: Embracing Your Desires

Write an Affirmation About Your Kinks: Create a positive affirmation that helps you embrace your desires without shame. For example, "My kinks are a natural part of who I am, and I embrace them as a source of pleasure and connection."

Educate Yourself: If you feel unsure about your kink or fetish, spend time learning about it. Understanding the psychology and safety behind your desires can help reduce feelings of shame and increase your confidence in exploring them.

Visualize Positive Exploration: Close your eyes and imagine a positive, respectful scenario in which you explore your kink or fetish with a partner. Visualizing the experience can help reduce anxiety and make you feel more comfortable when the time comes to discuss it openly.

Embracing and Exploring Kinks and Fetishes in a Healthy Way

Kinks and fetishes are a normal part of human sexuality, and learning to embrace them without shame can lead to deeper, more fulfilling sexual experiences. By communicating openly with your partner, setting clear boundaries, and exploring your desires in a safe and consensual manner, you can fully enjoy this aspect of your sexuality. Remember, there's no "right" way to express your desires as long as both partners feel respected, safe, and excited to explore together.

Chapter 11: Sexuality and Aging – Embracing Change and Finding Fulfillment

As men age, their sexual experiences and needs naturally evolve, often in ways they may not anticipate. Physical changes such as fluctuating testosterone levels, decreased stamina, and slower recovery times can impact sexual performance. However, these changes don't have to lead to dissatisfaction or a decline in sexual enjoyment. In fact, many men discover that aging can bring new opportunities for deeper emotional connections, a redefined sense of intimacy, and a broader understanding of what constitutes fulfilling sex.

This chapter explores how men's sexual experiences change as they move into their 40s, 50s, and beyond. We will also discuss how to adapt to these changes, strategies for maintaining satisfying sexual relationships, and how to embrace the emotional and mental aspects of sex that become even more vital with age.

Sex in Your 40s, 50s, and Beyond: How Sex Evolves as Men Age

The Impact of Aging on Male Sexuality

Aging is a natural process, and with it comes changes in the body's physical and hormonal makeup. Understanding how these changes affect sexual performance and libido is the first step toward adapting to a new, healthier perspective on sex in later life.

1. Declining Testosterone Levels

A gradual decline in testosterone levels is one of the most significant changes men experience as they age. Testosterone plays a key role in regulating libido, sexual performance, and overall energy levels. While the decrease in testosterone typically begins in a man's 30s, it becomes more noticeable as he enters his 40s and 50s.

<u>Effect on Libido</u>: Many men find that their sexual desire decreases as testosterone levels decline. This doesn't mean the end of a healthy sex life, but it does require adjusting to new rhythms of desire and arousal.

<u>Impact on Erections</u>: Testosterone is also linked to erectile function. As levels drop, men may experience changes in the strength or duration of their erections. These changes are normal but can sometimes lead to frustration or insecurity.

2. Physical Changes and Stamina

In addition to hormonal shifts, men also experience changes in physical fitness and stamina as they age. It's common for men to notice that they take longer to become aroused, need more time to recover between sexual encounters, or experience fatigue more quickly during sex.

<u>Longer Recovery Times</u>: Men may require more time between sexual encounters to feel ready for sex again. This is a normal part of aging and doesn't signal a decline in sexual ability, but rather a shift in how the body responds.

<u>Decreased Stamina</u>: Physical stamina can also decrease with age, affecting sexual endurance. Men may find that

they tire more easily or that their sexual pace naturally slows down, requiring more focus on foreplay and less emphasis on vigorous physical activity.

3. Changes in Erections and Ejaculation

It's also common for men to experience changes in their erections and the way their bodies respond during sex. Erections may not be as firm or as long-lasting, and ejaculation may take longer to achieve or feel less intense.

<u>Erectile Changes</u>: As blood flow decreases with age, men may experience softer erections or more difficulty maintaining an erection during intercourse. These changes are normal and can be managed through lifestyle adjustments or medical interventions if necessary.

<u>Delayed or Weakened Ejaculation</u>: Some men notice that ejaculation takes longer to achieve or is less forceful than when they were younger. This change can actually be beneficial for men who struggled with premature ejaculation in their younger years, as it allows for a slower, more controlled experience.

Exercise 1: Reflecting on Changes with Age

Write Down Physical Changes: List any changes you've noticed in your body or sexual function as you age. This can include libido, erections, stamina, or recovery time.

Reframe Your Perspective: Next to each change, write a positive aspect of your current sexual experiences. For example, while you may notice a decrease in stamina, you might find that you now take more time to enjoy the emotional aspects of sex.

Adapting to a New Sexual Pace: Keeping Satisfaction High as Your Body Changes

Shifting Your Focus

As physical changes occur, it's essential to adapt to a new sexual pace that aligns with your body's evolving needs. This adjustment doesn't have to detract from your sexual experiences—in fact, it can open the door to more mindful, emotionally fulfilling connections.

1. Embrace Slower, More Mindful Sex

As men age, sex often becomes more about quality than quantity. Slowing down and focusing on the emotional and physical sensations of sex can lead to a more satisfying and intimate experience. Instead of striving for the fast-paced, high-energy sex you may have enjoyed in your younger years, embrace a slower, more deliberate approach that emphasizes connection over performance.

Focus on Foreplay: With slower arousal and more time needed to build excitement, foreplay becomes an essential part of sexual encounters. Use this time to explore your partner's body, engage in sensual touch, and foster emotional intimacy. This shift toward prolonged foreplay can increase satisfaction for both partners.

Practice Mindfulness During Sex: Mindfulness—being fully present in the moment—can enhance sexual pleasure. Focus on the sensations you're experiencing rather than worrying about performance. Pay attention to touch, breath, and connection to your partner. This approach can deepen your emotional and physical bond.

2. Redefine What "Good" Sex Means

As you age, it's important to let go of the belief that "good" sex only involves frequent intercourse or intense orgasms. Redefine what satisfying sex means for you and your partner, focusing on connection, pleasure, and emotional intimacy rather than solely on the physical act of intercourse.

Expand Your Definition of Intimacy: Sexual intimacy doesn't always have to include penetration or orgasm. Kissing, cuddling, and non-sexual touch can all foster closeness and emotional connection, especially if your physical stamina or arousal levels fluctuate.

Let Go of Performance Pressure: Aging can bring greater emotional maturity and self-acceptance. Use this time to let go of performance pressure and focus instead on the joy of being with your partner, exploring each other's bodies, and deepening your emotional connection.

3. Adjust Expectations About Frequency

As men age, their need for frequent sex may decrease, which can be challenging for those who associate sexual frequency with virility or self-worth. Understand that having sex less often is a natural part of the aging process and doesn't diminish your masculinity or the health of your relationship.

<u>Quality Over Quantity</u>: Focus on the quality of your sexual encounters rather than how often they occur. Prioritizing emotional connection, meaningful touch, and mutual satisfaction can lead to more fulfilling sex—even if it happens less frequently.

<u>Communicate with Your Partner</u>: Open communication with your partner about changing sexual needs is vital. Ensure that you're both comfortable with the frequency and type of sex that occurs in your relationship. Discuss any concerns or adjustments that need to be made as your sexual rhythms evolve.

Embracing the Emotional Aspects of Sex as You Age

As men age, the emotional and relational aspects of sex often take center stage. While physical stamina or performance may change, emotional connection and intimacy can grow stronger, leading to deeper sexual satisfaction.

1. Emotional Intimacy Takes on Greater Importance

As men move into their 40s, 50s, and beyond, emotional intimacy often becomes more central to the sexual experience. Rather than focusing solely on physical

pleasure, many men find greater fulfillment in connecting
with their partner on a deeper emotional level.

Communication and Openness: Honest communication is
essential for building emotional intimacy. Sharing your
thoughts, fears, and desires with your partner can deepen
the emotional connection, making the physical aspects of
sex more meaningful and enriching.

Affection and Tenderness: As sexual intensity decreases,
affection and tenderness become increasingly important.
Expressing love, care, and appreciation through touch,
words, and gestures can deepen your bond and foster a
sense of closeness that goes beyond physical performance.

2. Sex as a Form of Emotional Connection

For many men, sex in later life becomes less about physical
release and more about emotional connection. The physical
act of sex becomes a way to reinforce emotional closeness,
trust, and partnership.

Bonding Through Touch: As your body changes, touch
becomes a powerful tool for maintaining emotional
intimacy. Non-sexual touch, such as holding hands,
hugging, or lying close to your partner, can reinforce your
emotional connection and enhance your overall relationship.

Sexual Intimacy as Emotional Reassurance: Sex can also
serve as a form of emotional reassurance, helping partners
feel desired, valued, and connected. Use sex as an
opportunity to affirm your love and commitment to your

partner, regardless of how your physical capabilities change.

3. The Role of Emotional Maturity

Aging brings with it emotional maturity and wisdom that can enhance your sexual experiences. With age, many men find that they are more patient, less focused on superficial aspects of sex, and better able to enjoy the emotional and relational components of intimacy.

Increased Self-Acceptance: As you age, you may become more comfortable with your body and your sexual desires. This increased self-acceptance allows you to let go of insecurities and focus on the deeper emotional connection with your partner.

Letting Go of Ego: Emotional maturity often involves letting go of ego-driven concerns about performance or sexual prowess. As you age, the need to "prove" yourself sexually diminishes, allowing you to focus more on mutual pleasure and connection.

Strategies for Maintaining Sexual Health and Vitality

While physical changes are inevitable, there are several strategies you can use to maintain sexual health, enhance performance, and enjoy a satisfying sex life well into your later years.

1. Stay Physically Active

Physical fitness plays a necessary role in maintaining sexual health. Regular exercise improves cardiovascular health, increases stamina, and promotes overall well-being—all of which contribute to a healthier sex life.

<u>Strength and Flexibility</u>: Strength training and flexibility exercises can help maintain muscle tone and range of motion, making sexual activity more comfortable and enjoyable.

<u>Cardiovascular Health</u>: Aerobic exercises such as walking, jogging, or swimming improve blood flow, which is essential for maintaining erections and overall sexual performance.

2. Eat a Healthy Diet

A balanced, nutrient-rich diet can support sexual health and vitality. Foods that promote heart health—such as fruits, vegetables, whole grains, and lean proteins—are also beneficial for maintaining healthy sexual function.

<u>Limit Alcohol and Processed Foods</u>: Excessive alcohol consumption and processed foods can negatively impact libido and sexual performance. Moderation is key to maintaining energy and stamina.

<u>Stay Hydrated</u>: Proper hydration supports overall physical health, including sexual health. Drinking plenty of water can help improve energy levels and stamina during sexual activity.

3. Manage Stress and Mental Health

Mental and emotional health play a significant role in sexual satisfaction. High levels of stress, anxiety, or depression can affect libido and sexual performance. Take steps to manage stress and prioritize your mental well-being.

<u>Practice Relaxation Techniques</u>: Techniques such as deep breathing, meditation, or yoga can help reduce stress and improve focus during sexual activity.

<u>Seek Professional Help If Needed</u>: If mental health challenges such as anxiety or depression are affecting your sex life, consider seeking the help of a therapist or counselor. Addressing these issues can lead to improvements in both emotional and sexual well-being.

Embracing Sexual Evolution with Age

Aging brings changes to the body, but it also brings wisdom, experience, and emotional depth that can make sex even more satisfying than it was in younger years. By adapting to a new sexual pace, prioritizing emotional intimacy, and embracing the changes that come with age, men can continue to enjoy fulfilling and rewarding sexual experiences throughout their lives. Remember, sexual satisfaction is not about chasing youthful performance—it's about deepening connection, fostering intimacy, and enjoying the emotional and physical pleasure that comes with a lifetime of growth.

PART V: Relationships, Power Dynamics, and Social Expectations

Relationships are complex and multi-faceted, especially when it comes to the dynamics of power, control, and societal expectations. These elements not only shape how individuals interact with each other but also influence how they express their desires, vulnerabilities, and boundaries within their intimate relationships. For many men, navigating these power dynamics can be especially challenging, as cultural and social norms often push rigid definitions of masculinity, dominance, and sexual performance.

This part of the book explores how men can build healthy, respectful, and mutually satisfying relationships by understanding and addressing power dynamics, questioning societal expectations, and fostering communication and consent. We'll examine how to approach power and control in sexual and emotional relationships and offer guidance for creating more balanced and equitable partnerships that empower both partners.

Chapter 12: Navigating Power Dynamics in Sex

Power dynamics—especially those involving sexual dominance and submission—can be an exciting and deeply rewarding aspect of many intimate relationships. For some men, the appeal lies in exploring different aspects of control, trust, and expression in a safe, consensual space. However, these dynamics are nuanced and require clear communication, well-established boundaries, and mutual consent to ensure both partners feel respected, understood, and secure throughout the experience.

In this chapter, we will explore why men are often drawn to power dynamics, how to navigate them in a way that honors control and mutual respect, and how to establish clear, healthy boundaries to ensure these dynamics remain safe and consensual. We will also address common misconceptions about dominance and submission, offering guidance on how to enjoy these experiences without fear of losing control or compromising one's values.

Sexual Dominance and Submission: Exploring the Appeal

Why Men Are Drawn to Power Dynamics

Sexual dominance and submission, also known as power play, involve one partner taking control while the other surrenders, often creating a heightened sense of pleasure and excitement. For many men, the appeal of these dynamics comes from stepping outside traditional roles and embracing an intense, raw form of connection. The allure of either dominating or submitting often allows men to explore different aspects of their personality, sometimes even aspects they may not express in their daily lives.

The Appeal of Dominance

Many men find the idea of dominance appealing because it taps into traditional ideals of masculinity, control, and leadership. Dominance in a sexual context involves taking charge, guiding the encounter, and often being responsible for a partner's pleasure. This role can be empowering, as it allows men to embrace their desire to lead and protect while also giving their partner the freedom to submit fully.

Escapism: For men who carry significant responsibilities in their daily lives, submission offers a chance to let go of control and escape the pressures of daily life.

Heightened Sensation: Power dynamics often amplify physical and emotional sensations, leading to more intense sexual experiences.

Masculinity and Control: For some men, dominance aligns with traditional masculine ideals that value strength, decisiveness, and control. In the bedroom, these traits can be explored in a way that is consensual and mutually pleasurable.

Responsibility for Pleasure: Many men enjoy the responsibility that comes with dominance, as it requires them to be attentive to their partner's needs and desires. This role can foster a deeper connection, as the dominant partner must be in tune with their submissive partner's emotional and physical cues.

Trust and Vulnerability: While dominance may seem like a position of power, it also requires vulnerability. The dominant partner must be willing to accept the responsibility that comes with control and be mindful of the trust their partner places in them. This dynamic can foster a deep sense of intimacy and mutual respect.

2. The Appeal of Submission

While dominance is often seen as the default expectation for men in traditional sexual roles, many men are equally drawn to submission. Submitting to a partner allows one to explore openness, relinquish control, and experience pleasure through trust and surrender. This allows for a different, yet equally fulfilling, dynamic within intimate relationships.

Relinquishing Control: For some men, the appeal of submission lies in the opportunity to relinquish control in a safe, consensual environment. In everyday life, men may be expected to be strong and in control, but submission offers a way to let go of those pressures and focus solely on receiving pleasure.

Emotional Intimacy: Submission can also foster emotional intimacy, as it requires a deep level of trust in the dominant partner. By submitting, men allow themselves to be vulnerable, which can strengthen their emotional connection with their partner.

<u>Freedom from Expectations</u>: Submission can offer freedom from societal expectations of masculinity. Men who submit can explore a different side of their sexuality, embracing the experience of being led, cared for, or even guided in ways that they might not normally experience.

The Psychology of Power Play

Power dynamics in sex often tap into deeper emotional and psychological needs. Dominance and submission go beyond physical acts, offering a chance to explore trust, openness, and emotional connection. When approached consensually and with clear boundaries, these dynamics can enhance intimacy and provide a safe space for exploring fantasies that may otherwise be challenging to express.

Exercise 1: Reflecting on Power Dynamics

Identify Your Desires: Write down any power dynamics you've fantasized about involving dominance, submission, or a combination of both. Be specific about what excites you about these dynamics.

Consider Emotional and Psychological Appeal: Reflect on why these dynamics appeal to you. Is it about control, trust, surrender, or something else? Understanding your motivations will help you approach power play with greater awareness.

The Fear of Losing Control: Challenging Traditional Masculinity

Power Dynamics and Masculinity

Traditional views of masculinity often emphasize control, strength, and stoicism. These cultural norms can create internal conflict for men interested in exploring sexual submission or even certain forms of dominance that involve vulnerability. For some, the idea of surrendering control in a sexual context may feel like a challenge to their sense of manhood or strength.

However, embracing power dynamics doesn't diminish masculinity—it expands it. The ability to be vulnerable (by submitting or trusting your partner to respect your boundaries) is an emotional strength. Similarly, when practiced consensually and respectfully, dominance can be about more than control—it can reflect leadership, care, and responsibility for your partner's well-being.

Breaking the Fear of Submission

For men who struggle with the idea of submitting, the fear often stems from a concern about how it reflects on their masculinity. Society teaches men to always be in control, but in a safe, consensual sexual context, letting go of control can be a deeply liberating experience. Submission is not a sign of weakness, but of trust and openness, allowing a partner to guide the experience.

Exercise 2: Exploring Control and Openness

Challenge Traditional Masculinity Beliefs: Begin by writing down any beliefs you hold about masculinity and control. For instance, do you believe that "real men" should always be in control or dominant? Reflect on these ideas and challenge them by considering how embracing openness, sharing control, or letting go of certain expectations could actually strengthen your relationships and deepen your sexual experiences. Explore how this shift might allow for more balanced, fulfilling connections.

Visualize Letting Go of Control: If submission interests you but feels intimidating, close your eyes and visualize a scenario in which you trust your partner to take control. Focus on the emotions of trust and freedom rather than fear. This can help you reframe submission as an empowering experience.

Healthy Dominance and Consent: Navigating Power Play Responsibly

The Importance of Consent and Communication

Power dynamics in sex—dominance or submission—rely heavily on mutual consent. Consent is the foundation of any healthy sexual relationship, but it becomes even more crucial when engaging in power play. Both partners must clearly express what they are comfortable with and where their boundaries lie. Power play is only enjoyable when both partners feel safe and respected.

Open and honest communication is the cornerstone of any healthy relationship, but it is particularly important in relationships that involve power dynamics. Both partners must feel comfortable discussing their desires, boundaries, and concerns before, during, and after exploring dominance and submission.

<u>Discuss Desires Openly</u>: Before engaging in power dynamics, it's essential to have an open conversation about what each partner is interested in. This includes talking about what dominance or submission means to each person, what activities are appealing, and what limits should be set.

<u>Use Clear, Direct Language</u>: Be specific in your communication. If you're interested in exploring dominance, make sure your partner understands what you mean by that. Are you interested in physical dominance, verbal commands, or emotional control? Clear language ensures that both partners are on the same page.

<u>Check in Regularly</u>: Communication doesn't end once the dynamic begins. It's important to check in with each other regularly throughout the experience. This can be done verbally or through pre-agreed non-verbal signals to ensure that both partners are comfortable and enjoying the experience.

2. Establishing Boundaries and Consent

Consent is non-negotiable in any sexual relationship, but it is especially important in dynamics involving power. Both partners need to agree on what is and isn't acceptable before engaging in dominance and submission, and they must respect each other's boundaries at all times.

Set Clear Boundaries: Before exploring power dynamics, have an honest discussion about your boundaries. Both partners should feel comfortable expressing what they are willing to do and what they are not. Boundaries should be respected at all times, and they can evolve as trust grows within the relationship.

Use Safe Words: Safe words are a critical tool for maintaining consent in power dynamics. These pre-agreed words allow a submissive partner to communicate when they need the activity to stop immediately. It's essential that the dominant partner respect the safe word and stop all activity as soon as it's used.

Respect the Right to Withdraw Consent: Consent is ongoing, and either partner has the right to withdraw consent at any time. If one partner becomes uncomfortable or wants to stop, their decision must be respected without question.

3. Respect and Trust

The foundation of healthy power dynamics is mutual respect and trust. Without these elements, dominance and submission can become abusive or manipulative. Both partners must feel valued, safe, and respected throughout the experience.

Mutual Respect: Regardless of whether you are the dominant or submissive partner, respect is paramount. The dominant partner must respect the submissive's boundaries and feelings, and the submissive must trust that the dominant partner will honor their limits and desires.

Build Trust Gradually: Power dynamics require a high level of trust, which should be built over time. Start slowly and experiment with different activities at a pace that feels comfortable for both partners. As trust grows, you can explore more intense or complex dynamics.

Navigating Power Dynamics Without Losing Control

Some men fear that exploring dominance or submission will lead to a loss of control—either over themselves or over the relationship. These fears are valid but can be mitigated through careful self-awareness and communication. Here's how to explore power dynamics without compromising your values or sense of self.

1. Understanding the Balance of Power

It's important to understand that power dynamics, even when one partner assumes dominance, are about balance and mutual agreement. True dominance isn't about controlling or overpowering your partner—it's about leading with care and responsibility.

Dominance as a Gift of Trust: When a partner submits, they are giving their trust to the dominant partner. This trust must be honored by ensuring that the submissive's well-being and pleasure are prioritized at all times. Dominance, therefore, becomes an act of responsibility, not coercion.

Submission as Empowerment: Submission doesn't mean losing power—it means willingly giving up control in a specific, consensual context. For many, the act of submitting can be empowering, as it allows them to trust their partner fully and embrace vulnerability.

2. Staying Grounded in Your Values

If you're concerned about losing control while exploring power dynamics, it's important to stay grounded in your values. Remind yourself that dominance and submission, when done consensually and respectfully, are expressions of mutual trust and love.

<u>Maintain Mutual Respect</u>: Respect is key, no matter the dynamic. If you feel that your actions do not align with your values, take a step back and reevaluate your approach. Dominance and submission should never involve humiliation, coercion, or manipulation unless both partners have explicitly consented to that dynamic.

<u>Be Mindful of Emotional Impact</u>: Power dynamics can evoke strong emotions for the dominant and submissive partner. Be mindful of how these dynamics affect your partner emotionally, and be open to discussing any concerns they may have.

3. Enjoying the Experience Without Fear

Exploring power dynamics should be a fulfilling and enjoyable experience for both partners. Let go of the fear of losing control or judgment and focus instead on the connection, trust, and excitement that come from exploring these dynamics safely and consensually.

Focus on Connection: Power dynamics can deepen emotional and physical connections between partners. Focusing on the bond you share with your partner allows you to enjoy the experience fully without fear of losing control.

Celebrate Vulnerability: Vulnerability is a key part of exploring dominance or submission; celebrate the fact that both partners are willing to open themselves up emotionally and physically in ways that foster intimacy and trust.

Healthy Dominance: Leading with Care

For men exploring sexual dominance, it's important to understand that healthy dominance isn't about control for control's sake—it's about creating an experience that is fulfilling for both partners. Dominance requires responsibility, attentiveness, and care for your partner's needs.

Healthy Dominance Involves:

Attuning to Your Partner: Being dominant means paying close attention to your partner's responses, both verbal and nonverbal. Always check in to ensure they enjoy the experience and feel comfortable.

Being Responsible: As the dominant partner, you ensure that boundaries are respected and that your partner feels safe throughout the encounter.

<u>Respecting Limits</u>: Even in a dominant role, it's essential to respect the agreed-upon boundaries. Dominance doesn't mean ignoring your partner's limits—it means guiding the experience within the boundaries of mutual consent.

Exercise 3: Establishing Boundaries for Power Play

Set Your Boundaries: Before engaging in any power dynamic, write down your boundaries—what you're comfortable with and what's off-limits. This clarity will make it easier to communicate with your partner.

Discuss Power Play with Your Partner: Have an open discussion with your partner about the dynamics you want to explore. Be transparent about your desires and encourage them to share theirs. Use this conversation to establish safe words, set limits, and ensure that both of you feel excited about the experience.

Exploring Power Dynamics Safely and Respectfully

Sexual dominance and submission offer men a unique way to explore their sexuality and masculinity. By embracing power dynamics consensually, men can enhance their sexual relationships and experience new depths of intimacy and trust. The key to healthy power play is clear communication, mutual respect, and an unwavering commitment to consent.

Remember, power dynamics are not about control or domination in the negative sense—they are about creating a space for shared pleasure, trust, and emotional connection. By navigating these dynamics responsibly, you can enrich your sexual experiences and build stronger, more intimate relationships with your partner.

□

Chapter 13: The Social Pressure to Be a "Sexual Performer"

Today, men are constantly bombarded with messages about what it means to be a "real man" in bed. From movies and pornography to casual conversations and cultural norms, the pressure to be a perfect sexual performer—always dominant, always in control, and always delivering satisfaction—can create a narrow and often harmful view of male sexuality. These unrealistic expectations can lead to feelings of inadequacy, anxiety, and disconnection from the true essence of sex: connection, pleasure, and mutual enjoyment.

This chapter will explore how societal myths about male sexuality shape our understanding of what it means to be a man in the bedroom, the harmful impact of these pressures, and how to reclaim a more authentic, healthy, and fulfilling approach to sex by redefining masculinity in the bedroom.

Societal Myths About Male Sexuality

The pressure to be a "sexual performer" comes mainly from societal myths and outdated ideas about masculinity. These myths perpetuate rigid expectations of men as sexually dominant, always ready for sex, and capable of delivering endless satisfaction to their partners. While these ideas are widely promoted in popular culture, they fail to represent the reality of human sexuality and place unnecessary pressure on men to meet impossible standards.

1. The Myth of Constant Readiness

One of the most pervasive myths is that men are always ready and willing for sex. This idea suggests that a "real man" should have an unending sexual appetite, be able to perform on command, and never turn down an opportunity for sex. This myth ignores the natural fluctuations in desire that everyone experiences and sets men up for feelings of inadequacy when their libido doesn't match these unrealistic expectations.

Reality Check: Sexual desire is not constant and is influenced by many factors, including stress, emotional state, physical health, and relationship dynamics. It's completely normal for desire to ebb and flow. Men shouldn't feel pressured to always be "in the mood" to prove their masculinity.

2. The Myth of Performance-Based Worth

Another damaging myth is that a man's worth is tied to his sexual performance. This idea suggests that men must be skilled in bed, able to last for long periods of time, and consistently bring their partner to orgasm to be considered sexually competent. This places immense pressure on men to focus on performance over connection, often leading to anxiety, stress, and a disconnection from their own pleasure.

<u>Reality Check</u>: Good sex is about mutual pleasure, connection, and communication—not about achieving a specific outcome. Men are not defined by their ability to meet certain performance standards. True sexual satisfaction comes from emotional intimacy, exploring desires together, and enjoying the experience.

3. The Myth of Sexual Dominance

Society often glorifies the idea of men as sexually dominant, taking charge in the bedroom and controlling the sexual experience. While some men may enjoy dominance as part of consensual sexual dynamics, this myth can make men feel inadequate if they prefer a more equal or even submissive role in sexual encounters. It also reinforces the idea that men must be aggressive or in control to be sexually desirable.

<u>Reality Check</u>: Sexual dominance isn't the only expression of masculinity. Every man has the right to express his sexual desires in a way that feels authentic and pleasurable to him, whether that involves being dominant, equal, or even submissive. Mutual consent and exploration of different dynamics are what matter most.

The Myth of the Alpha Male: Society's Pressure on Men to Perform Sexually

The idea of the "alpha male" is one of the most pervasive and damaging stereotypes men face when it comes to sexual performance. According to this myth, the "ideal" man is always dominant, always in control, and always ready for sex. He's expected to have unshakable confidence, perform for extended periods, and please his partner in every conceivable way. This image not only creates unrealistic expectations but also places an enormous burden on men to meet a performance standard that is neither sustainable nor necessary for a fulfilling sexual relationship.

Key Elements of the Alpha Male Myth:

<u>Dominance</u>: Men are often expected to take the lead and maintain control in sexual encounters.

<u>Endurance</u>: There's an assumption that men should have endless stamina and that anything less is a failure.

<u>Perfection</u>: The idea that a man must always satisfy his partner, leaving no room for mistakes.

<u>Always Ready</u>: Men are taught that they should be ready for sex at any moment and should feel embarrassed if they aren't.

The Harmful Impact of Performance Pressure

The pressure to meet these societal expectations can have a profound impact on men's sexual experiences, emotional well-being, and relationships. When men feel that they must live up to unrealistic ideals, it can lead to anxiety, self-doubt, and even disconnection from their own pleasure and their partner's.

1. Performance Anxiety and Sexual Dysfunction

One of the most common consequences of performance pressure is performance anxiety—the fear of not being able to live up to expectations in the bedroom. This anxiety can manifest as erectile dysfunction, premature ejaculation, or difficulty achieving orgasm, as the pressure to perform interferes with the natural sexual response.

<u>Erectile Dysfunction (ED)</u>: When men are preoccupied with the fear of not being able to maintain an erection or satisfy their partner, it can lead to performance-related erectile dysfunction. The anxiety and stress of needing to perform "perfectly" can prevent men from relaxing and enjoying the moment.

<u>Premature Ejaculation (PE)</u>: For some men, the pressure to perform can lead to premature ejaculation. The overwhelming focus on delivering pleasure or proving one's masculinity can cause men to rush the sexual experience, unable to relax and control their arousal.

2. Emotional Disconnection and Loss of Pleasure

When men are focused solely on performance, they often lose touch with the emotional and physical pleasure that sex is meant to bring. Instead of enjoying the moment and connecting with their partner, they become hyper-focused on achieving certain goals—such as lasting longer, making their partner orgasm, or maintaining an erection—which can lead to a disconnection from their own desires.

<u>Disconnection from Partner</u>: The pressure to perform can make men feel distant from their partner, as they may be too focused on fulfilling a role rather than enjoying the

experience together. This can create emotional distance and reduce intimacy in the relationship.

<u>Disconnection from Self</u>: Constantly worrying about performance can cause men to lose touch with their own pleasure. Rather than focusing on what feels good for them, they may prioritize their partner's satisfaction or their own ability to meet societal standards, leading to a loss of enjoyment in sexual experiences.

3. Strained Relationships

The performance pressure men experience can also create tension in their relationships. When sex becomes a source of anxiety or stress, it can affect communication, emotional closeness, and overall relationship satisfaction.

<u>Unspoken Expectations</u>: When men feel pressured to perform, they may avoid discussing their needs, fears, or insecurities with their partner, leading to a lack of open communication about sex. This can create unspoken expectations that go unmet, causing frustration for both partners.

<u>Reduced Intimacy</u>: When sex becomes focused on performance, the emotional and physical intimacy that comes with sexual connection can be diminished. This can leave both partners feeling unsatisfied, even if the sexual experience appears "successful" from the outside.

Exercise 1: Challenging the Alpha Male Myth

List the Pressures You Feel: Write down the specific pressures or expectations you feel when it comes to sex. Are you worried about lasting long enough, being dominant, or always being ready? Acknowledging these pressures is the first step in breaking free from them.

Challenge Each Pressure: Next to each pressure, write down why it's unrealistic or unnecessary. For example, "I don't always have to be in control during sex—sometimes, sharing the lead can be more satisfying and intimate."

Reclaiming Your Sexuality: Moving Beyond Performance to Connection and Pleasure

Sex Isn't About Performance

One of the biggest misconceptions men face is that sex is a performance to be measured. In reality, sex is a shared experience rooted in pleasure, connection, and mutual respect. It's not about how long you last, how many times you can perform, or how dominant you are—it's about how you and your partner feel during and after the experience.

To break free from the harmful impact of societal pressure, men must learn to redefine masculinity in the bedroom and embrace a more authentic, healthy approach to sex. This involves letting go of the need to perform and focusing on mutual pleasure, connection, and emotional intimacy.

1. Redefining Masculinity in the Bedroom

True masculinity in the bedroom is not about dominance, control, or meeting arbitrary performance standards. Instead, it's about being present, communicating openly with your partner, and enjoying sex as a shared, mutual experience.

<u>Focus on Connection, Not Performance</u>: Shift your mindset from performing for your partner to connecting with them. Focus on how the experience feels rather than what you're achieving. Pay attention to your partner's emotional and physical responses and allow yourself to be vulnerable in the moment.

<u>Embrace Emotional Intimacy</u>: Real sexual satisfaction comes from emotional closeness and trust. Be open with your partner about your fears, desires, and insecurities. When you allow yourself to be vulnerable, you create space for a deeper emotional connection that enhances sexual intimacy.

<u>Prioritize Mutual Pleasure</u>: Sex should be a mutually enjoyable experience. Instead of worrying about your own performance, focus on what feels good for both you and your partner.

2. Communicating Openly with Your Partner

Open communication is key to breaking free from performance pressure. Talk to your partner about your needs, desires, and any anxieties you may have about sex. This conversation can help to foster understanding, relieve pressure, and make sex a more fulfilling experience for both of you.

<u>Discuss Your Expectations</u>: Have an honest conversation about the expectations you feel when it comes to sex. This

can help dispel myths about what sex "should" look like and give both partners a clearer understanding of each other's desires.

Share Your Insecurities: Don't be afraid to share any insecurities you have about your sexual performance. Being open about these feelings can reduce anxiety and allow both partners to support each other.

3. Focusing on Mutual Pleasure and Exploration

Sex is about mutual pleasure and exploration, not about achieving a specific outcome. By focusing on the journey rather than the destination, men can let go of performance pressure and rediscover the joy of sexual connection.

Explore Together: Try new things together in the bedroom without focusing on if they're "successful" or not. Experiment with new positions, take your time with foreplay, or talk more openly about your fantasies; the goal is to enjoy the process rather than aiming for a specific result.

Practice Mindful Sex: Mindfulness can help you stay present during sex, reducing anxiety and helping you focus on physical sensations and emotional connection. Practice being fully in the moment, paying attention to your partner's touch, breath, and responses.

How to Reclaim Pleasure in Sex

To break free from the performance-driven mindset, it's important to reconnect with what sex is truly about pleasure. This involves slowing down, being present in the moment, and allowing yourself to enjoy the experience without focusing on meeting certain expectations.

Ways to Reclaim Pleasure:

<u>Slow Down</u>: Take your time during sex. Enjoy the sensations, the intimacy, and the connection with your partner. Rushing to a finish line only reinforces the idea of sex as a performance.

<u>Let Go of Outcomes</u>: Release the pressure to meet specific goals, like achieving an orgasm or maintaining an erection for a certain amount of time. When you focus on enjoying the experience itself, performance anxiety often disappears.

Exercise 2: Reclaiming Pleasure in Your Sexual Experiences

Reflect on Past Experiences: Think about times when sex felt like a performance. What were you focused on? Was it pleasure and connection, or achieving a certain outcome? Write down any patterns you notice.

Focus on Pleasure in Your Next Encounter: The next time you're intimate with your partner, focus entirely on the sensations and emotions you're feeling in the moment. Don't worry about how long you last or if you're "performing" well. Instead, focus on enjoying the connection.

Embracing a New Vision of Sexuality

The pressure to be a "sexual performer" is a heavy burden that many men carry, but it doesn't have to define your sexual experiences. By letting go of the alpha male myth, reclaiming your sexuality as something rooted in connection and pleasure, and redefining masculinity in a more holistic way, you can enjoy a healthier, more fulfilling sex life.

Sex is not about performing for someone else's approval—it's about sharing an intimate, pleasurable experience with your partner. When you embrace open communication and mutual enjoyment, sex becomes a richer, more satisfying part of your life.

Chapter 14: Embracing Vulnerability and Openness

At the core of sexual self-awareness is the willingness to embrace vulnerability. In a world that often glorifies invulnerability and control, being vulnerable can feel risky or uncomfortable, especially when it comes to sex. Yet, true intimacy and growth come from the ability to open yourself up emotionally and mentally, allowing you to connect with your partner—and yourself—on a deeper level.

1. Vulnerability Is Strength

Society often teaches men that showing vulnerability, especially in the context of sex, is a sign of weakness. However, being vulnerable requires courage and strength. It's through vulnerability that you can truly express your desires, fears, and insecurities, which opens the door to genuine connection and understanding. In embracing vulnerability, you foster deeper emotional intimacy with your partner, allowing both of you to feel seen, understood, and supported.

<u>Emotional Openness</u>: When you express your true emotions—love, desire, fear, or insecurity—you create a safe space for your partner to do the same. This emotional transparency enhances the quality of your relationship, building a foundation of trust that strengthens your bond.

<u>Breaking Down Barriers</u>: By letting go of the need to always appear in control or perform to a certain standard, you allow yourself to break down internal barriers that may

have been holding you back from fully enjoying sexual intimacy.

2. Communication as the Foundation of Growth

Open and honest communication is one of the most powerful tools for cultivating sexual self-awareness. When you communicate your desires, boundaries, and needs, you not only strengthen your relationship with your partner but also enhance your understanding of your own sexuality. Communication goes beyond simply discussing preferences—it's about fostering an ongoing dialogue where both partners feel heard and respected.

<u>Creating Comfortable Dialogue</u>: Both you and your partner should feel comfortable discussing any aspect of your sexual relationship without fear of judgment. This creates an environment where you can openly explore your desires and navigate any challenges or insecurities together.

<u>Listening with Compassion</u>: Being open to listening—truly listening—can deepen your understanding of your partner's needs and desires, allowing you to support one another in your sexual and emotional growth.

Staying Curious and Embracing Growth

Sexual self-awareness is an ongoing journey. There's no finish line, no ultimate destination to reach where you know everything there is to know about sex or yourself. Sexuality evolves throughout your life, and what you desire, enjoy, or need at one stage may change over time. By maintaining a mindset of curiosity and openness, you can continue to grow, adapt, and discover new dimensions of your sexual self.

1. Explore Without Judgment

As you explore your sexuality, it's important to let go of judgment—self-judgment or the fear of being judged by others. Everyone's sexual journey is unique, and there's no "right" way to experience or express desire. By allowing yourself to explore your fantasies, preferences, and curiosities without shame, you can create a more authentic relationship with your sexuality.

Experimenting Together: With your partner, explore new things that excite you—a new activity, fantasy, or conversation about desires. This exploration can strengthen your bond, as both of you are given the freedom to express yourselves without judgment.

Learning and Growth: Sexuality is a lifelong process of learning. Continue seeking out resources—books, articles, workshops, or conversations with your partner—that help you grow in your understanding of yourself and your relationship. Stay curious about how your body, emotions, and mind work together to create fulfilling sexual experiences.

2. Reevaluate Your Desires and Needs Over Time

As life changes, so do your desires and needs. Your sexual experiences in your 20s may look different from those in your 40s, 50s, and beyond. As you age, your priorities and preferences may shift, and it's essential to embrace these changes rather than resist them. Sexual self-awareness involves regularly checking in with yourself and your partner to ensure that you're both satisfied and fulfilled in your evolving sexual lives.

<u>Adapt to Changes</u>: Be open to adapting and evolving to physical changes related to aging, emotional shifts in your relationship, or newfound interests in exploring new facets of your sexuality. Growth often comes from change and embracing it can lead to new and exciting experiences.

<u>Celebrate Every Stage</u>: Every stage of life offers something new regarding sexual discovery. Celebrate the lessons you've learned, the experiences you've had, and the deeper emotional connections you've fostered. By appreciating the evolution of your sexuality, you cultivate a healthier and more satisfying sexual life.

Cultivating Compassion for Yourself

As you continue on your journey toward greater sexual self-awareness, it's imperative to practice compassion—both for yourself and for your partner. Sexuality is deeply personal, and it's easy to be hard on yourself if things don't go as expected or if you feel insecure about certain aspects of your sexual life. However, true growth comes from understanding that mistakes, insecurities, and challenges are all part of the process.

1. Let Go of Perfectionism

There's no such thing as "perfect" sex, nor should that be the goal. Instead of striving for an idealized version of sexual success, focus on the pleasure, connection, and fulfillment that each experience brings. Every sexual encounter—whether it goes smoothly or not—is an opportunity to learn more about yourself and your partner.

Focus on the Experience: Let go of the pressure to perform or meet expectations, and instead focus on being present in the moment. The best sexual experiences are often those that prioritize emotional and physical connection over performance.

2. Be Kind to Yourself

It's natural to feel insecure or anxious at times when it comes to sex, but don't let these feelings define you. Be kind to yourself when things don't go as planned, and remember that every experience offers an opportunity for growth.

Celebrate Small Wins: Every step you take toward greater self-awareness, either communicating more openly with your partner or exploring a new aspect of your sexuality, is worth celebrating. Recognize your progress and give yourself credit for the work you're doing.

Embracing the Journey

Sexual self-awareness is not a destination; it's a lifelong journey. It's a path of exploration, growth, and deepening connection with yourself and others. Along this journey, there will be moments of discovery, challenges to overcome, and opportunities for transformation. By staying open to new experiences, embracing vulnerability, and practicing compassion, you can continue to cultivate a fulfilling, satisfying, and authentic sexual life that evolves with you.

Remember, there's no rush—no finish line to cross. Your journey is unique, and the only measure of success is how connected, fulfilled, and confident you feel in your sexuality. Keep asking questions, keep learning, and keep embracing the wisdom of your own sexual self-awareness.

Conclusion: Embracing the Wisdom of Sex

As we've explored throughout this book, having more wisdom about sex is a powerful tool that empowers men to break free from societal pressures, deepen their connections, and foster healthier, more satisfying relationships. It's a journey that involves vulnerability, curiosity, and a willingness to challenge traditional norms. In this conclusion, we'll discuss the importance of open conversations about sex, the ongoing nature of sexual growth, and practical next steps to continue your journey toward greater self-awareness and fulfillment.

The Power of Open Conversations

Breaking Taboos and Asking Questions

One of the most important steps toward sexual wisdom is the ability to talk openly about sex. For too long, men have been conditioned to avoid discussing their desires, fears, or insecurities, which only deepens feelings of shame or confusion. By encouraging open dialogue—with a partner, a trusted friend, or a therapist—men can begin to break down the barriers that hold them back.

Why Open Conversations Matter:

<u>Destigmatizing Taboo Topics</u>: Many aspects of male sexuality are still considered taboo, from emotional vulnerability to issues like erectile dysfunction or sexual fluidity. The more men talk openly about these topics, the less power the stigma has over them.

Building Deeper Connections: Open conversations foster trust and emotional intimacy, both in sexual and non-sexual contexts. This deepens relationships and helps partners better understand each other's needs.

Learning Through Dialogue: Asking questions and sharing experiences with others allows men to learn and grow. No one has all the answers, but by engaging in honest conversations, you can gain valuable insights into your sexuality and relationships.

Exercise 1: Start a Conversation

Identify a Trusted Person: Choose someone in your life who you trust and feel comfortable discussing personal matters with. It could be a partner, friend, or therapist.

Start Small: Initiate a conversation about a sex-related topic that you've been curious about or hesitant to discuss. This might be about your desires, body image, or a challenge you've faced. Starting small can help build confidence for future discussions.

Sex as a Lifelong Journey

Understanding the Evolution of Sexual Wisdom

Sexuality is not static—it evolves as we age, as our relationships change, and as we grow emotionally. The wisdom you gain from your sexual experiences will continue to develop over time, bringing new challenges and opportunities for personal growth. What matters is not

achieving some final "goal" of sexual mastery but embracing
the journey of continual learning, experimentation, and self-
awareness.

Key Aspects of the Sexual Journey:

Adapting to Change: Understanding that sex will evolve
over time. Aging, changing desires, or shifting dynamics in
relationships allows you to stay open to new experiences
and approaches.

Embracing Imperfection: There's no such thing as perfect
sex. Some encounters will be great, others might not go as
planned, and that's okay. What's important is how you grow
from each experience.

Staying Curious: Keep asking questions, exploring new
dynamics, and learning from your partners and yourself.
Curiosity is the key to long-term sexual fulfillment.

Exercise 2: Reflect on Your Sexual Growth

Look Back: Take some time to reflect on how your
understanding of sex and sexuality has changed over the
years. What have you learned, and how have you grown?

Look Forward: Consider areas of your sexuality that you'd
like to explore or understand better. Write down a few ways
you can continue to grow in the future—learning,
conversation, or experience.

Next Steps: Practical Resources for Continued Learning and Growth

As you move forward in your journey toward sexual wisdom, it's essential to continue seeking knowledge, support, and personal growth. There are many resources available to help you navigate different aspects of sexuality, from educational materials to professional support networks.

The Wisdom of Sex– A Lifelong Journey of Growth and Connection

Wisdom of sex is about far more than improving performance or mastering specific techniques. It's a path toward deeper understanding—of yourself, your desires, your boundaries, and your emotions. Sexuality, much like every other aspect of life, is a lifelong process of growth, discovery, and evolution. As you continue this journey, it's important to remember that sexual fulfillment isn't achieved by conforming to societal expectations or hitting predetermined milestones. Instead, it's found in the ongoing pursuit of self-discovery, emotional connection, and open communication with both you and your partner.

This journey is about fostering a healthy relationship with your sexuality—free from guilt, shame, or unrealistic expectations. It's about embracing curiosity, being vulnerable, and understanding that every step, no matter how small, is progress toward greater self-awareness and fulfillment.

Recommended Resources for Continued Learning:

<u>Books on Sexuality</u>: Consider exploring books that offer other insights into topics like sexual health, intimacy, and relationship dynamics. Some recommended reads include:

- Come as You Are by Emily Nagoski (exploring sexual desire and arousal)
- The New Male Sexuality by Bernie Zilbergeld (addressing men's sexual issues and solutions)
- The Ethical Slut by Dossie Easton and Janet W. Hardy (for those exploring non-monogamy and open relationships)

<u>Therapy and Counseling</u>: If you're facing challenges around sexual issues like anxiety, body image, or relationship dynamics, seeking help from a therapist can provide valuable guidance. Many therapists specialize in sex therapy or couples counseling.

<u>Workshops and Classes</u>: Look into workshops, classes, or retreats that focus on sexual health, intimacy, and personal growth. These can provide hands-on learning and help you connect with others on a similar journey.

<u>Support Networks and Online Communities</u>:

- <u>Online Forums and Support Groups</u>: Engage with online communities where men discuss their experiences, ask questions, and offer support. Reddit's "r/MensLib" or "r/Sex" can be good starting points for non-judgmental discussions.

- <u>Sexual Health Websites</u>: Trusted websites like, The Kinsey Institute, and Goop's Sex and Relationships section offer a wealth of information on various sexual health topics.

Dr. Wisdom's YouTube Channel

https://www.youtube.com/@thewisdomof

Bonus Section 1: Frequently Asked "Unaskable" Questions

In this section, we tackle some of the most common but rarely asked questions about sex that many men are too embarrassed or afraid to bring up. Dr. Wisdom provides honest, straightforward answers to help you better understand your body, mind, and sexual experiences.

Q1: Is it normal to not always want sex?

Answer: Absolutely. The idea that men should always be in the mood for sex is a harmful stereotype. Libido can fluctuate due to stress, health, emotional connection, or simply the natural ebb and flow of desire. It's important to communicate openly with your partner and not feel pressured to perform on demand.

Q2: Why do I sometimes lose my erection during sex?

Answer: Losing an erection is more common than you might think and can happen for a variety of reasons, including stress, anxiety, fatigue, or even a lack of emotional connection at the moment. It's important to approach this with self-compassion rather than panic. If it becomes a recurring issue, consider discussing it with a doctor or therapist to rule out physical or psychological causes.

Q3: Is it normal to have fantasies about other people, even if I love my partner?

Answer: Yes, having fantasies about others doesn't mean you're unhappy in your relationship. Fantasies are a natural part of sexual imagination and don't always reflect real desires. It's important to differentiate between fantasy and reality and to communicate with your partner about what excites you without feeling guilty.

Q4: How do I deal with performance anxiety?

Answer: Performance anxiety is often linked to unrealistic expectations or pressure to "perform" a certain way. To combat this, focus on being present in the moment, communicate openly with your partner, and shift your mindset from outcome-based goals to enjoying the experience. Mindfulness techniques, breathing exercises, and reducing external pressures can also help ease anxiety.

Q5: Why does my sex drive seem lower than it used to be?

Answer: There are many factors that can affect libido, including age, stress, lifestyle, hormonal changes, and relationship dynamics. It's important to pay attention to your physical and mental health. If the change is concerning, consider speaking with a healthcare professional to explore potential causes, such as low testosterone or mental health issues.

Q6: How do I talk to my partner about a kink or fantasy I'm afraid they'll judge me for?

Answer: Open communication is key. Start by creating a safe, non-judgmental space for conversation, and gently introduce the idea by expressing it as something you're curious about exploring together. Be prepared for your partner's reaction, and make sure to discuss boundaries. It's important to approach the conversation with respect, understanding, and patience.

Bonus Section 2: Sexual Health Checklist for Men

Maintaining sexual health isn't just about physical performance—it's about taking care of your overall well-being, including mental and emotional health. Here's a comprehensive checklist to help you stay on top of your sexual health.

1. Regular Medical Check-ups

<u>Annual Physical Exams</u>: Regular check-ups with your doctor can help catch any health issues early, including conditions that may affect sexual function, like diabetes or heart disease.

<u>Blood Pressure and Cholesterol</u>: High blood pressure and cholesterol can impact circulation, which affects erectile function.

<u>Testosterone Levels</u>: If you notice a drop in libido or energy, ask your doctor about getting your testosterone levels checked, especially as you age.

2. Sexual Health Screenings

<u>STI Screenings</u>: Regular screenings for sexually transmitted infections (STIs) are important, especially if you have new or multiple partners. Many STIs are

asymptomatic, so don't assume you're in the clear without testing.

<u>Prostate Health</u>: As men age, prostate health becomes increasingly important. Speak with your doctor about prostate screenings, especially after age 50.

3. Mental Health and Stress Management

<u>Therapy and Counseling</u>: Mental health is closely linked to sexual health. Anxiety, depression, and stress can all impact libido and performance. If you're struggling, consider speaking with a therapist who specializes in men's mental health or sexual issues.

<u>Mindfulness and Relaxation</u>: Incorporating mindfulness practices, meditation, or breathing exercises into your routine can help reduce stress and improve sexual performance.

4. Diet and Exercise

<u>Healthy Diet</u>: A balanced diet supports overall health, including sexual function. Focus on foods that promote good heart health, like fruits, vegetables, lean proteins, and whole grains.

<u>Regular Exercise</u>: Staying physically active improves blood circulation, stamina, and confidence. Cardiovascular exercises, in particular, can enhance sexual performance.

5. Communication and Relationship Health

<u>Open Dialogue</u>: Regular, honest conversations with your partner about your sexual desires, concerns, and needs are critical for maintaining a healthy sexual relationship.

<u>Emotional Intimacy</u>: Building emotional intimacy with your partner can deepen your connection and improve your sexual experiences. Take time to nurture your relationship outside of the bedroom.